Anatomy and Physiology for Veterinary Technicians and Nurses

A Clinical Approach

Website

This book is accompanied by a companion website:

www.wiley.com/go/sturtz

The website includes:

- The figures from the book for downloading into PowerPoint
- Additional questions and answers
- Labeling quizzes
- Teaching PowerPoints
- A dissection video

Anatomy and Physiology for Veterinary Technicians and Nurses

A Clinical Approach

Robin Sturtz, DVM
Associate Professor, Associate Director, Veterinary Technology Program, Mercy College, Dobbs Ferry, NY
Associate Veterinarian, The Cat Hospital, Williston Park, NY

Lori Asprea, LVT
Bachelor of Science, Mercy College

Ilustrations by Robin Sternberg, LVT

WILEY-BLACKWELL
A John Wiley & Sons, Inc., Publication

This edition first published 2012 © 2012 by John Wiley & Sons, Inc.

Wiley-Blackwell is an imprint of John Wiley & Sons, formed by the merger of Wiley's global Scientific, Technical and Medical business with Blackwell Publishing.

Editorial offices: 2121 State Avenue, Ames, Iowa 50014-8300, USA
The Atrium, Southern Gate, Chichester, West Sussex, PO19 8SQ, UK
9600 Garsington Road, Oxford, OX4 2DQ, UK

For details of our global editorial offices, for customer services and for information about how to apply for permission to reuse the copyright material in this book please see our website at www.wiley.com/wiley-blackwell.

Library of Congress Cataloging-in-Publication Data
Sturtz, Robin.
Anatomy and physiology for veterinary technicians and nurses : a clinical approach / Robin Sturtz,
Lori Asprea.
p. cm.
Includes bibliographical references and index.
ISBN 978-0-8138-2264-8 (pbk. : alk. paper)   1. Veterinary anatomy.   2. Veterinary physiology.
I. Asprea, Lori.   II. Title.
SF761.S87 2012
636.0892–dc23
2012012163

A catalogue record for this book is available from the British Library.

Wiley also publishes its books in a variety of electronic formats. Some content that appears in print may not be available in electronic books.

Set in 10/12 pt Minion by Toppan Best-set Premedia Limited
Printed and Bound in Singapore by Markono Print Media Pte Ltd

Disclaimer

1   2012

Dr. Sturtz would like to thank LVTs Asprea and Sternberg and dedicates this book to her students, teachers, family and pets, which should about cover it.

Lori Asprea (coauthor, photography) thanks her mother and father, sister, and entire family; Mercy College and the Vet Tech Department; and, of course, Robin Sturtz and the animals. Without them, this book would be very boring. I would like to dedicate this book to my family, who has endlessly supported my ambitions.

Robin Sternberg (illustrations) thanks Drs. Jennifer Chaitman, Anthony Pilny, and Eveline Han, and would like to dedicate this book to Dr. Jennifer Chaitman—my mentor, my friend, and my inspiration.

Contents

Companion website

This book is accompanied by a companion website:

www.wiley.com/go/sturtz

Preface

The authors and the illustrator have all been students as well as teachers of veterinary science. We have long talked about putting together a book that reflects how we think about the subjects of anatomy and physiology. For one thing, we sought to have the anatomy and the physiology portions of the book as two separate sections. In some veterinary technology programs, anatomy and physiology are actually taught as separate courses. Even when they are combined, it can be more helpful to build on the foundation of a complete understanding of the anatomy in order to understand the complexity of physiology.

We all agree that adding clinical scenarios makes the information more interesting and, thus, easier to remember. Anatomy and physiology are not part of our curriculum for the sake of theory. The aim of the study of these topics is to be able to apply this knowledge to daily practice in a clinic, hospital, or research facility.

In this first edition, there are materials that have no doubt been excluded that might have been included, or concepts that were included but do not strike the readers as interesting to the same level that the authors find them to be. We fervently hope that this work will be of use. We hope equally as much that you, the reader, will let us know what information you would like added or subtracted as we move forward. Please note that any errors are solely the responsibility of Dr. Sturtz.

We hope that you find this book worthwhile, not only for current study but also for frequent reference. There are also online components that will be of help for people who learn best with visual images rather than written narrative.

Robin Sturtz
Lori Asprea

Acknowledgments

It is absolutely impossible to write and illustrate a book like this without the support and guidance of dozens of people. It is possible to go on for pages of excruciating detail thanking everyone who has helped us with this project. However, in deference to the reader, we shall endeavor to be brief.

The guidance of our teachers has sustained us and carried us to this moment. We thank the faculty and staff at all of the colleges we have attended (the authors have Mercy College in Dobbs Ferry, New York, in common). We thank our family and friends for their tremendous forbearance. We particularly thank our students for their enthusiasm, their patience, and their encouragement, not to mention their perfect timing when it comes to asking that one last question . . .

Our good friends at John Wiley & Sons are, of course, the ones who made this all happen. To Nancy and all of the editorial wizards there, our deepest gratitude.

Dr. Sturtz would like to honor a few special people: Professors Buell, Burke, and Burke at Mercy College; Drs. C. Brown, S. Brown, P. Carmichael, and S. Allen at The University of Georgia College of Veterinary Medicine; friends and colleagues at La Guardia Community College, Mercy College, and The Cat Hospital; the veterinary Bregman family; Kim, Ceasar, Judy, Glen, and Jon, and a whole host of others. Kudos to Elaine Sturtz for last-minute artwork. (Yay mom!) If I've met you, count yourself in.

And, of course, we all thank our pets, who could probably write this book just as well as we did, but who preferred to sit back and laugh at us while we did it. Good going, pets!

R.S.
L.A.

Anatomy and Physiology for Veterinary Technicians and Nurses

A Clinical Approach

SECTION 1
ANATOMY

Chapter 1 Directional Terms

Clinical case: Fluffy

A veterinary technician comes in for work in the morning to discover that Fluffy has come in overnight after having been hit by a car. The chart note indicates that there is "a cut on the back leg." This, of course, gives very little information.

The study of anatomy is, put simply, the study of the structure of organisms. It involves looking at architecture, at the different positions, shapes, and sizes of various living tissues. As one might imagine, the anatomy of different species has some things in common and some things that are quite diverse. The structure of the heart is very similar in dogs and cats; it is quite different in equines and reptiles. The kidneys of the dolphin look very different from those of the dog, although they function in the same way. By understanding the differences in anatomy among animals, we can have a greater appreciation for how their body systems function. This understanding is the basis of recognizing states of health and disease.

There are a number of different ways to organize how one looks at anatomy. Gross anatomy refers to features that can be seen with the naked eye. Developmental anatomy is the study of how anatomy changes as the fetus becomes a puppy or a kitten. Topographic anatomy refers to the relation to the parts to the whole (e.g., how the different parts of the kidneys and the connecting conduits make up the urinary system). Regional anatomy refers to the structures of a given area of the body; if one looks at the head, for example, as one unit, it would involve the study of all the muscles, blood vessels, bones, and other tissues that are present. Imaging anatomy refers to the anatomical features as they are seen on a good radiograph. Applied anatomy refers to the anatomy that is most important surgically or for medical treatment. In planning orthopedic surgery, for instance, it is necessary to know not only the structure of the bones but also the local muscles and blood vessels. Most of us use a systems approach. We study all of the bones, then all of the muscles, then all of the digestive organs, without regard to where they are placed.

One of the most important issues in studying anatomy is the understanding of directional terms. If one is asked to find a particular spot on the animal, having someone say "It's on the leg" is not terribly precise. Saying that a spot is "just proximal to the right stifle" (just above the right knee) is much clearer. While the acquisition of vocabulary can be tedious, it is the way to communicate clearly with our clients, veterinarians, and other members of the patient-care team. In other words, good anatomic vocabulary contributes to excellent patient care.

Anatomy and Physiology for Veterinary Technicians and Nurses: A Clinical Approach, First Edition. Robin Sturtz and Lori Asprea.
© 2012 John Wiley & Sons, Inc. Published 2012 by John Wiley & Sons, Inc.

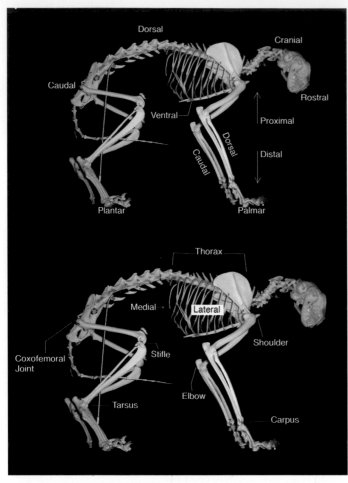

Figure 1.1   Directional terms as they pertain to the feline/canine skeleton. Also noted are some of the major joints.

thorax. The areas around the ribs are referred to as costal areas. The abdomen refers both to the outer surface (the skin) of the ventrum and also to the space within it. The thoracic inlet is the area of the ventral thorax where the neck ends.

The space within the thorax is called the thoracic cavity, and the space within the abdomen is the abdominal cavity. Note, however, that some of the features of each of these are lined by a membrane. The pleural membrane, within the thorax, surrounds the lungs and lines the walls of the thoracic cavity. The area bordered by this membrane is considered to be within the pleural cavity. Similarly, the membrane surrounding some of the organs and lining the interior walls of the abdomen is the peritoneal membrane, or peritoneum, and that space is called the peritoneal cavity. Inflammation of that membrane is called peritonitis. There is a viral disease called feline infectious peritonitis that causes inflammation of the peritoneum (among other things). The localized inflammation is so severe that a condition called ascites (fluid in the abdomen) can result. This disease is incurable and can only be treated symptomatically.

Features of the limbs get special names. The front legs are referred to as the thoracic limbs, the rear legs as the pelvic limbs. The shoulder and elbow in dogs are, in medical terms, the scapulohumeral and humeroradioulnar joints, respectively. The next joint distal to the elbow is the carpus, the equivalent of the human wrist. The front of the leg from the shoulder going distally to the paw is the dorsal section, with the back of that area up to the carpus referred to as the caudal section of the limb. On the pelvic limb, the joint between the femur and the tibia is the femorotibial joint, commonly known as the stifle; it is equivalent to the human knee. The next joint going distally is the tarsus. The common name for the tarsus is the hock. The same terms, dorsal and caudal, apply to the pelvic limb.

The part of the thoracic limb from the shoulder to the elbow is referred to as the brachium; the area from the elbow to the carpus is the antebrachium. The area from the head of the femur (the proximal-most bone of the pelvic limb) to the stifle is called the femoral area. The area from the stifle to the tarsus technically is called the crus, although that term is not commonly used in a clinical setting; distal pelvic limb is less precise but often used in general practice.

There is one other directional label referring to the limbs. The area from the carpus distally, on the caudal surface, and around to and including the ventral surface of the paw, is known as the palmar surface. The analogous area from the tarsus to the bottom of the paw is the plantar surface.

The joints of equines have a number of common names that are distinct from those of small animals. For example, the carpus is called the knee, and the tarsus is called the hock.

There are different names for the bones themselves in large animals. The long bone distal to the carpus and tarsus is known as the cannon (equivalent to the third metacarpal/metatarsal bone of dogs and cats). The three bones of the digit, called proximal, middle, and distal phalangeal bones, have a different set of names. They are called, respectively, long pastern, short pastern, and coffin bone. We will discuss the specific names of bones in Chapter 3.

Directional terms in veterinary medicine are very different from those used in human medicine. The human head is "up" from the hips, while it is "forward" in the dog. This is another reason that it is important to use the proper terms.

Going toward the head is considered to be cranial; going in the opposite direction is caudal. Going from the floor upward is traveling in a dorsal direction. From the top downward is moving in a ventral direction. On the limbs, we use special terms. Closer to the body is proximal; going away from it is moving in a distal direction (Figure 1.1).

Moving toward the center is going medially. Going out from the midline to the side of the animal is a lateral movement. On the head, there is a special term. When we discuss something that is cranial to another spot on the head, we describe it as rostral (from the Latin word for face).

We need to add some more vocabulary to refer to specific places. The part of the body that includes the chest and abdomen is referred to as the trunk. The proper name for the ventral part of the abdomen is the ventrum. The proper name for the top of the trunk is the dorsum. The lateral surface of the part of the trunk caudal to the chest is the flank.

There are specific names for other parts of the body. The part of the trunk from the neck to the caudal ribs is referred to as the

Clinical case resolution: Fluffy

In the example at the beginning of this chapter, a problem was noted with Fluffy's "back leg." The chart note is not terribly precise. We can record that Fluffy has a laceration proximal to the right stifle, on the medial surface of the limb, and it will be clear to any reader exactly where the problem is. This is the advantage of using correct anatomical terms.

Review questions

1 Define the terms medial, rostral, and dorsal.
2 Which is more cranial, the thoracic limb or the pelvic limb?
3 The caudal paw area on the thoracic limb is referred to as the _____ surface.
4 True or false: The stifle is caudal to the tail.
5 Define the term "topographic anatomy."

Chapter 2 The Common Integument

Clinical case: Cat with alopecia

A cat is brought into the clinic for a general checkup and vaccines. There is an area of alopecia (missing hair) that is perfectly round. It is located on the dorsal surface of the animal's head and is about 0.5 cm in diameter. The skin is not irritated, and the client does not report that the cat has been scratching it.

The term integument refers to a broad range of tissues. Knowing the composition and structure of these elements contributes to a broader understanding of the function of this system. This will lead to the ability to recognize what happens in disease states such as the one described above.

Introduction

The integument is a collective term for aspects of bodily structure that are formed of connective tissue and epithelia. Connective tissue is a collection of proteins, fibrous material, and ground elements that form a great many parts of the mamma-lian body. An epithelial cell has a specific microscopic structure. Features such as skin, skin glands, fur/whiskers, hooves, horns, and claws are epithelial structures that are parts of the integument. This chapter will focus on mammals; certain species-specific characteristics will be discussed at the end of the chapter.

Skin

Mammalian skin has several layers to it. The superficial-most layer is the epidermis. Deep to it is the dermis. There is a layer of fat and connective tissue deep to the dermis called the subcutaneous layer. The subcutaneous layer is not skin (subcutaneous means below the surface of the skin) but is a part of the integument.

The epidermis itself has a number of layers. The deepest of these is the stratum basale. Continuing toward the surface, the layers are the stratum spinosum, stratum granulosum, stratum lucidum, and stratum corneum. See Figure 2.1 for a depiction of these layers.

Some parts of the epidermis have more layers than others. For example, there is no stratum lucidum in areas where there are hair follicles, or where the skin is very thin. In areas where

Anatomy and Physiology for Veterinary Technicians and Nurses: A Clinical Approach, First Edition. Robin Sturtz and Lori Asprea.
© 2012 John Wiley & Sons, Inc. Published 2012 by John Wiley & Sons, Inc.

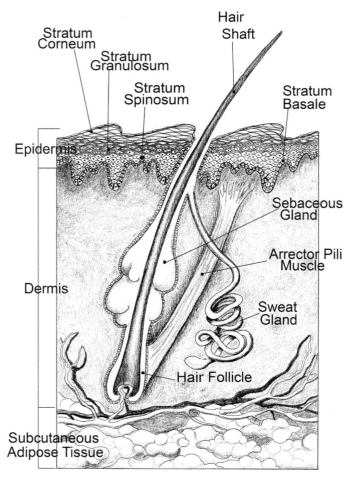

Figure 2.1   Layers of the skin. The epidermis ends at the stratum basale, and the dermis ends at the subcutaneous layer.

glands are found. It is a layer that has primary importance in the functions of skin as well as in structural support.

Dermal glands fall into two main categories: sweat and sebaceous. Sebaceous glands produce sebum, which is a waxy, thick substance. Sebaceous glands also secrete pheromones, which are species-specific odors that have a great deal to do with socialization and reproductive behaviors. There are a number of sebaceous glands throughout the body, in all mammalian species. The interdigital glands are important in ruminants. These are present in the area of the hoof where the digits begin to spread out from each other. The anal glands, present on either side of the anus, assume an important communication role in dogs and cats and will become quite familiar in clinical practice. Suborbital glands, present in the area of the medial canthus (place where the eyelids meet) of each eye, are used to mark territory by many antelopes.

Sweat glands are of two types, apocrine and eccrine. These types differ in their function and will be discussed in Chapter 14. In general, apocrine sweat glands are found in association with hair follicles, while eccrine glands are spread in other areas. Canines and felines have sweat glands primarily around the metacarpal and digital pads of the paw. A specialized form of sweat gland is the mammary gland.

A discussion of the skin would not be complete without a discussion of the subdermal or subcutaneous layer (usually abbreviated as "sub-Q" or "SQ"). This layer is mostly composed of adipose tissue (i.e., fat). When a cat or a dog picks a neonate up by the back of the neck, it is not painful. This is because she is holding him/her by the scruff. The scruff is the part of the body on the dorsal neck that has a very thin layer of skin, and is mostly composed of subcutaneous fat. Sub-Q, like the epidermis, has little in the way of blood vessels or nerve fibers. In a healthy animal, this layer has a large water content; in a dehydrated animal, areas of thick subcutaneous tissue, such as the scruff, will maintain a tented appearance if pinched and released, rather than springing back to a normal position. This is one way we assess hydration status during a physical examination.

Pads

A thickened mass of epidermal layers is referred to as a pad (see Figure 2.2). Dogs and cats have a pad on the palmar/plantar surface of each digit and a larger pad proximal to it called a metacarpal or metatarsal pad, depending on the limb (carpal always refers to the thoracic limb and tarsal to the pelvic limb). There is also a small pad in cats just proximal to the carpus. This pad is usually associated with one of the skin glands and is often marked by a single tactile hair.

Horses have pads on the limbs, referred to as the chestnut and ergot. The chestnut is found on the medial surface, in the area of the carpus/tarsus. Interestingly, chestnuts are thicker in working horses than in light breeds, where they may be absent altogether. The ergot is on the caudal surface in the same area as the chestnut on each limb. A concentration of sebaceous glands in this area may be involved in scent marking.

skin is thick, such as the specialized epidermis known as the pads of the paw and limb, there may be a relatively thick stratum lucidum.

The stratum lucidum and stratum corneum (from the Latin root for "horn") are composed of cells that are, for lack of a better word, dead. When the living cells are formed in the deepest layers of the epidermis, they work their way up toward the surface, dying along the way. By the time they reach the most superficial layer of the epidermis, the stratum corneum, they have lost their nuclei and are ready to slough off. These compose the flakes of "dry skin" that are noted on gross observation.

The epidermis has almost nothing in the way of blood vessels or nerve fibers. This is why a cat's head can be gently scratched without drawing blood. Anything that penetrates down to the level of the dermis, however, will cause pain and bleeding, as that is where the blood vessels and nerves are located.

The dermis is mostly composed of collagen, a protein. The bases of individual hairs are encased in a space called a follicle; the majority of the follicles lie within the dermis. The dermis is also where the nerves and blood vessels run and where the skin

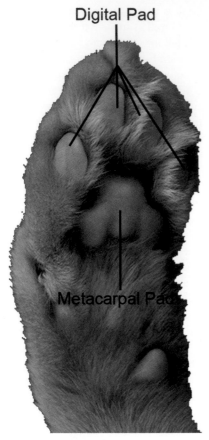

Digital Pad

Metacarpal Pad

Figure 2.2   Pads of the feline paw.

Haircoat

The haircoat is an important feature of the integument. One of the attributes that defines an animal as a mammal is that it has hair.

In dogs and cats, the haircoat has several layers. The word topcoat is used to denote the outermost layer. The trapping of air between the coat and the undercoat is an important method of thermoregulation (see Chapter 14 for a further discussion of thermoregulation). The undercoat is usually thicker than the topcoat and is the layer that does most of the shedding. When a dog or cat is combed, it is mostly the undercoat that comes off onto the comb. The topcoat is composed of guard hairs. The hairs of the undercoat are referred to as wool hairs.

The whiskers (vibrissae) are a type of hair called tactile hair. They are thicker than guard hairs and are only present at certain places on the body; in mammals, they tend to cluster on the face. They sense motion and objects and should never be trimmed unless medically necessary.

There are some breeds of cats and dogs that are "hairless." The adjective is a misnomer in that they usually have whiskers and often at least some body hair. These animals suffer from a high incidence of skin cancer and problems with thermoregulation. Careful counseling of clients with these animals is important, particularly regarding the use of sunscreen and the treatment of dry skin.

Note that hairs die as they grow toward the surface, just as epidermal cells do. These dead structures are said to be keratinized, as they are filled with the protein keratin.

Claws

The claw is another type of epidermal tissue, and it is also composed of keratin. In some animals, including cats and dogs, there is often a digit with a claw on the medial surface of the limb called a dewclaw. The dewclaw does not make contact with the ground under normal circumstances and is vestigial. Dogs usually have a dewclaw on all four limbs. Cats, on the other hand, rarely have a dewclaw on the pelvic limbs. As a result, cats with 19 digits are considered to be polydactyl (having more than the normal number of digits). Polydactyl animals need to be observed carefully in relation to the growth of the claws. All claws, particularly those that do not make contact with the ground, may grow so long that they impinge on the pad and can cause pain or even infection if not monitored for length.

Given that they are composed of keratin, there is no pain associated with trimming the claws themselves. However, there is a vein associated with the distal phalanx (distal-most bone in the digit) that is visible at the base of the claw. Cutting it can cause significant pain and bleeding. Accidentally impinging on this vessel is called "cutting the quick," and is something to be avoided.

Onychectomy, commonly called "declawing," which is performed on cats under some conditions, involves removing the distal phalangeal bone (P3) as well as the claw itself. Failing to remove sufficient material can lead to regrowth of the claw; removing P3 as well ensures that this does not happen. (A fuller discussion of the bone structure of the paw will be found in the next chapter.)

Species differences

Feathers are actually a specialized type of epidermis and can be thought of as the haircoat of the avian (see Figure 2.3). The contour feathers are the outer layer, giving the bird its silhouette. The down feathers are deep to the contour feathers and tend to be smaller and more tufted. Clipping a bird's wings actually means trimming the longest contour feathers (primary flight feathers) back to the level of the shorter (secondary) flight feathers. This prevents the bird from flying long distances.

Hooves, horns, and beaks are also composed of epidermis. Thus, their outer surface is composed of "dead" tissue. This is why beaks and hooves can be trimmed without drawing blood (if done properly). Avian and reptile claws are epidermis as well and also can be trimmed.

The hoof has several layers, or laminae, which have an important function in ambulation. Basically, the laminae (layers) interdigitate, forming an interlocking series of tissues. Inflammation between those layers can lead to a very painful condition called laminitis, one of the most frustrating causes of equine lameness; it is, unfortunately, a common problem in equines and often

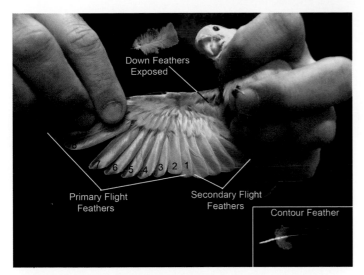

Figure 2.3 Types of feathers. "Clipping" a bird's wings refers to trimming the primary feathers so that the bird cannot fly too high or too far if housed in a restricted area. Contour feathers are the outermost ones, giving the body its outline. Down feathers are closest to the body and provide good insulation.

leads to intractable pain. The severity of the problem occasionally necessitates euthanasia.

While the cranial and caudal surfaces of the hoof are tough epidermis, the plantar/palmar surfaces are softer. Landmarks on this surface include the pad itself, known as the frog, and the sole, which takes up the majority of the ventral surface of the hoof.

Horn is also epidermis. In some species (e.g., ruminants), the horn actually fits over the skull such that there is a space running through the center of the horn and down into the frontal sinus of the skull. This is important from a husbandry standpoint. If the animal is to be dehorned, and proper procedure is not followed, any contamination at the base of the horn can lead to sinus infection. Lapses in aseptic technique can be associated with encephalitis, or inflammation of the brain. Both sinusitis and encephalitis are difficult to treat at best.

The difference between horn and antler is that antlers are shed and horns are usually not. In cervids, the antler is covered by a layer of softer epidermis called velvet, which eventually dies and falls away. The antler is shed after that point.

Clinical case resolution: Cat with alopecia

The cat in the case described at the beginning of this chapter has a condition called dermatophytosis, commonly known as "ringworm." Dermatophytes are a type of fungus that feed off keratin. Since the tissue they eat is dead, dermatophyte infections generally are not pruritic (itchy) and do not cause significant inflammation. They do, however, cause the hair to fall out in a circle around the area where the organisms are. It is a very common problem in cats, and to some degree in dogs, in the United States. Ringworm is important to know about because it is zoonotic. For that matter, it can also be passed to animals by humans.

Review questions

1 An animal has a laceration that is bleeding, but the cut does not extend down to the muscle. What layers of skin are involved?
2 List three examples of sebaceous glands.
3 Do cats sweat?
4 What organism is responsible for ringworm infection?
5 Of the following areas, where would the stratum lucidum of the epidermis be the thickest?
Eyelid
Lip
Digital pad
6 What is laminitis?
7 What is the difference between guard hairs and tactile hairs?
8 What is the difference between horns and antlers?
9 Which of the following is not painful?
Laminitis
Cutting the quick
Ringworm
10 What is meant by clipping a bird's wings?

Chapter **3** Skeletal Anatomy

Clinical case: Newborn puppy

A newborn puppy is brought into the hospital. He has been having difficulty nursing and seems to have milk running out of his nose right after a meal. He sometimes coughs while nursing.

Introduction

The study of the skeleton is the study of the framework of the animal's body. Invertebrates such as insects may have an external skeleton. The skeleton of the dogfish is mostly cartilage.

This discussion will concentrate on mammalian skeletons, which are mostly composed of bones. While there are small interspecies differences, the general features are the same. Mammalian skeletons are internal.

The structure of bones falls into a few main categories: long, short, flat, irregular, and sesamoid. Their growth patterns differ

to some extent. Long bones and flat bones are often used as a site for bone marrow sampling, for the purpose of laboratory analysis. Long bones and irregular bones have features with specific names (see Figure 3.1).

The skeleton is traditionally divided into two parts: axial and appendicular. The axial skeleton is considered to be the skull and vertebral column, including the caudal (tail) vertebrae. Some experts also consider the ribs and sternum to be part of the axial skeleton. Everything else is appendicular (literally, hangs from or is ventral to the axial skeleton).

The long bones

Long bones have cylindrical bodies, with a round or plateau-like end. The rounded area at the proximal end is referred to as the head, and at the distal end as a condyle. Condyles usually come in pairs and are generally described as medial or lateral. It is clear that it is not sufficient to say "the lateral condyle" as that can refer to a number of locations. It is always necessary to reference the landmark to the specific bone, as in "the lateral condyle of the humerus" (see Figure 3.2).

Anatomy and Physiology for Veterinary Technicians and Nurses: A Clinical Approach, First Edition. Robin Sturtz and Lori Asprea.
© 2012 John Wiley & Sons, Inc. Published 2012 by John Wiley & Sons, Inc.

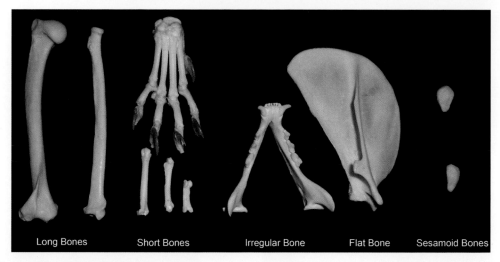

Figure 3.1   Types of bones. The sesamoid bones shown here are the patellae, which are located in the patellar tendon. The short bones are taken from the paw (shown intact above it).

Long Bones   Short Bones   Irregular Bone   Flat Bone   Sesamoid Bones

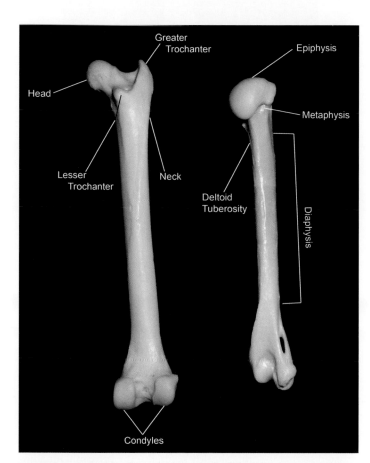

Figure 3.2   Features of long bones (on the left is the femur, on the right the humerus).

The shaft of the bone is referred to as the diaphysis. The proximal and distal surfaces are referred to as the epiphysis. The relatively short area between the epiphysis and the diaphysis of the bone is the metaphysis. These different areas have distinct growth patterns. In fact, there is a cartilaginous plate that separates the

metaphysis from the epiphysis, which is known as the physis (epiphyseal plate). This plate ossifies as the animal ages.

The superficial diaphysis and metaphysis are covered by a fibrous lining called periosteum. This covering contains blood vessels and nerve fibers. The vessels enter a pinpoint opening into the diaphysis called a nutrient foramen. The diaphysis has an interior tunnel that runs through it called a medullary cavity. The lining of that cavity is called endosteum. Bone marrow is located within the medullary cavity.

Long bones often have a rather wide projection called a trochanter. The best-known trochanter is the greater trochanter of the femur. A tuberosity is a smaller, often narrow ridge or projection. A stylus is a narrow, pointed projection at the distal end of a bone. A foramen is a hole. A fossa is a shallow depression on the surface of the bone (Figure 3.3). A process is also a projection from a bone, usually having a cone or peg shape. The neck of a long bone, as might be imagined, is the slightly narrow area just distal to the head of the bone.

The limbs contain most of the long bones of the body. The first ones we will discuss are those of the thoracic limb.

The thoracic limb

Conventionally, the scapula is considered to be a part of the limb because it is connected via the shoulder joint to the leg. The scapula forms the shoulder (scapulohumeral) joint in association with the humerus. The scapula is considered a flat bone. It does, however, have some additional geometry. The lateral surface of the scapula has a long, thin projection called the spine of the scapula (see Figure 3.4). It should be palpable on examination of the living animal. The ventral-most part of the spine of the scapula is called the acromion, which is important as a muscle attachment. The shallow depressions dorsal and ventral to the spine of the scapula are the supraspinous and infraspinous fossae, respectively. The fossa on the distal end of the scapula, into which the head of the humerus fits, is called the

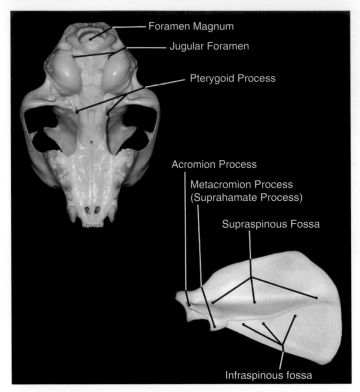

Figure 3.3 Views of the ventral skull and lateral scapula, showing features named fossa (plural is fossae), foramen (foramina), and process (processes). Note that the suprahamate process is found only in cats.

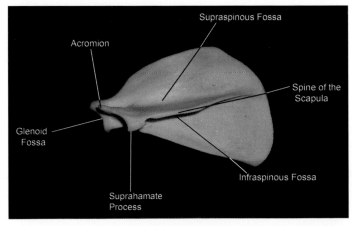

Figure 3.4 Landmarks of the scapula.

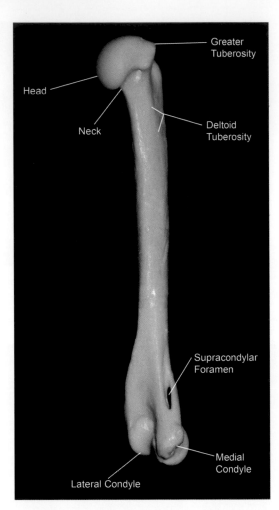

Figure 3.5 The humerus. Note that cats have a foramen to the medial side of the bone, called the supracondylar foramen; in dogs, this opening is in the center, between the condyles, as pictured here. It is called the supratrochlear foramen.

glenoid fossa. It is noteworthy that the scapula in cats and dogs is not directly attached to the rest of the skeleton; the only thing that holds it in place is muscle. Among other things, it means that it is easier to amputate the thoracic than the pelvic limb (such as in cases of malignancy) as no bony connections need be severed.

The humerus is the proximal-most long bone of the thoracic limb (see Figure 3.5). The humerus is distinguished by a head, a greater tuberosity, and a neck at its proximal boundary. The head of the humerus is a common site to sample bone marrow in cats.

The humerus has a structure called the deltoid tuberosity on its medial surface, which is the attachment for the deltoid muscle. The distal humerus has two condyles, a lateral and a medial. In dogs, there is a trochlear foramen between the condyles. In cats, the equivalent is the supracondylar foramen, which is on the medial surface of the bone and proximal to the condyles rather than between them.

The humerus meets up with the radius and ulna at a joint that is referred to as the radiohumeral joint, and is commonly called the elbow. The radius actually crosses over the cranial surface of the ulna from the medial to the lateral side, while the ulna is situated so that it points slightly medially. The proximal ulna has a number of specific features of importance (see Figure 3.6). The olecranon is the part that projects caudally (or caudodorsally, depending on the position of the limb) and is clearly palpable when examining the leg during an office visit. Going distally, there is a C-shaped structure called the trochlear notch. The proximal tip of it is called the coronoid process, and the distal tip is called the anconeal process. There is a congenital abnormality in some dogs known as ununited anconeal process, which

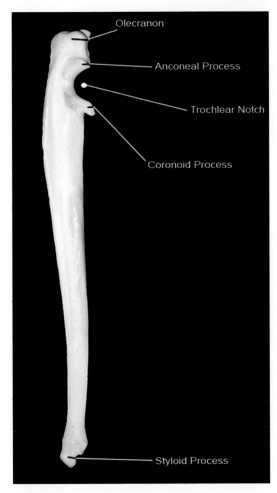

Figure 3.6   The ulna.

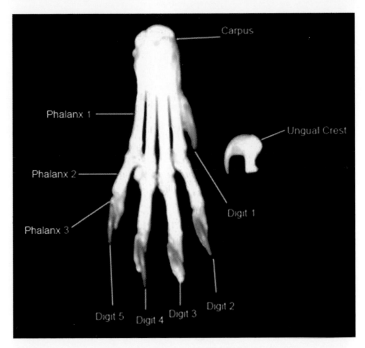

Figure 3.7   The digits of the paw are counted from medial to lateral as numbers 1 through 5. Digit number 1 is the dewclaw. The ungual crest is where the claw joins the distal-most bone of the digit.

is difficult to diagnose, but is associated with lameness. There is a styloid process on the medial surface of the distal ulna.

The joint distal to the elbow is the carpus, which is made of a series of short bones. Distal to those are bones that have been characterized as either flat or long bones, called the metacarpal bones. There is one for each digit. It is important to note that the metacarpals, and for that matter the digits, are numbered from the medial to the lateral side. In other words, the lateral-most digit in the dog and cat is number five. The dewclaw, which does not normally come in contact with the ground, is number one (see Figure 3.7).

The digits are a special case in that they are made of three bones in dogs and cats (usually only two in the dewclaw), at least one of which is irregular in shape, and one is short. Caudal to the metacarpophalangeal joints (the joints between the metacarpus and the proximal phalangeal bones) are small sesamoid bones, which help reduce tension on the tendons and ligaments of the paw.

The bones of the digits are called the proximal, middle, and distal phalangeal bones. They are often referred to as P1, P2, and P3, going distally. The distal part of P3 has a shallow fossa with a collar referred to as the ungual crest. It is here that the claw attaches to the digit (Figure 3.8).

Dogs may have dewclaws on all four limbs. Cats usually have dewclaws only on the thoracic limbs. Polydactyly is common in the dewclaw particularly, which is to say that there occasionally is more than one dewclaw on a given limb. It should be noted that pigs and some ruminants also have dewclaws.

The practice of removing the dewclaw was commonly done for hunting dogs. It was felt that the dewclaw could catch on the bushes and warn the prey animal that dogs and humans were in the area. Hunting dogs also often underwent docking, the removal of the distal tail, and cropping, the shortening of the pinna. Cropping was also done in show dogs. These procedures are illegal in Europe.

The pelvic limb

Unlike the thoracic limb, the joint where the pelvic limb connects to the body does, in turn, connect to the rest of the skeleton. As a result, the pelvic limb is considered to begin at the proximal-most long bone, which is the femur (see Figure 3.9). The femur is the longest bone in the dog and cat skeleton. It is distinguished by a large head, which fits into the coxofemoral (hip) joint. It has a prominent feature called the greater trochanter, which is on the lateral surface. It should be readily palpable on physical exam of the living animal. The distal end of the femur has a lateral and a medial condyle. The joint that is between the femur and the next most distal bone is the stifle joint; although the joint is properly called the femorotibial joint, the term stifle is universally used. It is incorrect to refer to this joint as the knee, as the knee in equines is actually the common name for the carpus, and confusion could easily result.

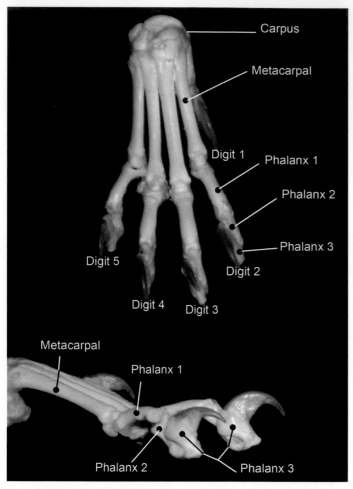

Figure 3.8   Cranial and lateral views of metacarpal and phalangeal bones. Lateral view shows a dewclaw and two digits.

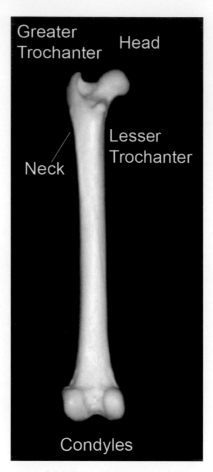

Figure 3.9   Features of the femur (left femur, caudal view).

The bone distal to the stifle is the tibia (see Figure 3.10). The tibia has a plateau-like proximal surface; the small peak in its center is referred to as the intercondylar eminence. On its cranial surface, it has a projection called the tibial tuberosity. These landmarks are important in discussing surgery of the stifle joint, particularly involving cruciate ligament disorders.

One of the most striking characteristics of the stifle is the patella, which is actually contained within a tendon (the tendon of insertion of the quadriceps). It is the largest of all the sesamoid bones in mammals; its shape is considered to be like that of a sesame seed, which is where the entire category of these bones gets its name.

Running parallel to the tibia is the fibula, a thin bone that sits next to the tibia's lateral surface. In equines and ruminants, this bone is actually fused to the tibia and is incomplete in its length. In dogs and cats, it ends along with the tibia at the next joint, the tarsus. This joint is made of a series of short and irregular bones. The tarsus has two irregular bones of note. One is the talus, which is rounded, and the other is the calcaneus, which is rectangular. The calcaneus is particularly important as the distal attachment for the gastrocnemius muscle, called the calcanean tendon; in humans, this is known as the Achilles tendon.

Distal to the tarsus are the metatarsal bones, distal to which are the digits. These bones are arrayed and numbered as they are in the thoracic limb. The exception, as mentioned, is that most cats do not have a dewclaw on the pelvic limbs.

Flat bones

The pelvis

The pelvis is known as the os coxae (see Figure 3.11). Although it appears to be one large bone, it is actually composed of three flat bones that are fused during fetal development. The pelvis is considered part of the appendicular skeleton.

The cranial-most section is known as the ilium. The cranial part of the ilium sweeps dorsally and is called the wing of the ilium. A dorsocranial section of the wing is called the ileal crest and is important as an area from which we take bone marrow samples in dogs. (In cats, the bone is too thin, and the head of the humerus is used more often for this.)

The ischium is the section caudal and ventral to the ilium. It is a relatively short section but is important because it accommodates a fossa known as the acetabulum. This area is where the

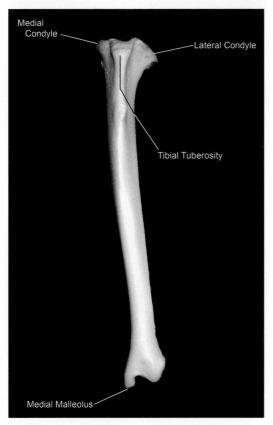

Figure 3.10   The tibia, cranial view. Note that the tibial tuberosity is an important surgical landmark.

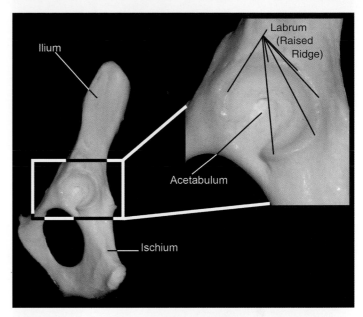

Figure 3.12   View of the pelvis with acetabulum magnified to reveal the labrum.

head of the femur sits, forming the coxofemoral joint. Fracture of the ischium, therefore, is often associated with hip joint problems. It should be noted that the acetabulum actually contains overlapping sections of the ilium, ischium, and pubis. Abnormalities of the acetabulum or of the head of the femur are part of hip dysplasia, which is a common orthopedic problem in large-breed dogs (see Figures 3.12 and 3.13).

The caudal part of the pelvis is the pubic bone. The pubis and the ischium together make up the borders of the obturator foramen, a large opening that is an important landmark.

The skull

The skull is composed mostly of flat bones (see Figures 3.14–3.16). The cranium is the part of the skull that contains the brain. The jaw is composed of a single bone ventrally, called the mandible. The mandible has a dorsoventral projection at its caudal end that is called the ramus. It is the only part of the mandible that does not have teeth. The dorsal jaw is made of two bones that fuse together during development but is generally referred to by one name, the maxilla. Technically, the maxilla is the part that encompasses the lateral surface of the dorsal jaw. The rostral point of the upper (maxillary) jaw is composed of a small bone called the incisive bone, which holds the small teeth known as incisors.

The entire skull is made of a series of flat bones that eventually meet and become one structure. This happens during fetal development. Occasionally, when the dorsal plates of the skull have not completely come together at birth, there is a small spot on the dorsal cranium that is left with no bony covering. This is called a fontanel. It should close shortly after birth. It can allow significant damage to the brain by traumatic injury if it remains open.

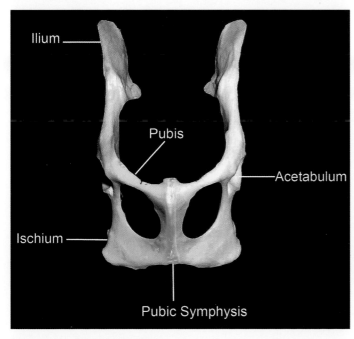

Figure 3.11   Bones of the pelvis.

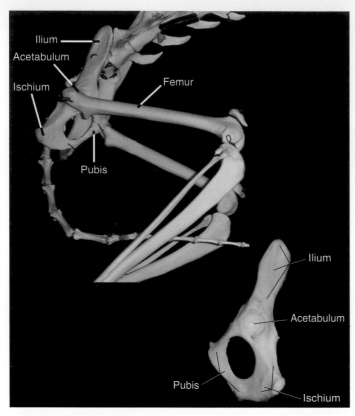

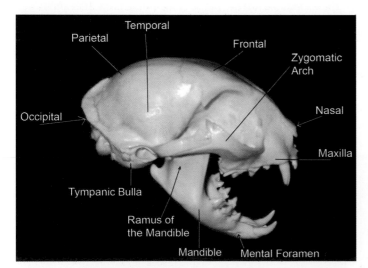

Figure 3.13   Lateral view of the pelvis and femurs (top). Bones of a halved pelvis (bottom).

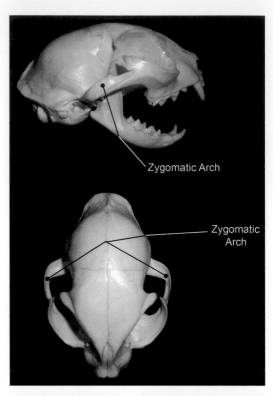

Figure 3.15   Views of the zygomatic arch. The caudal portion (indicated on the upper photo) is an extension of the temporal bone. The rostral portion is the zygomatic bone.

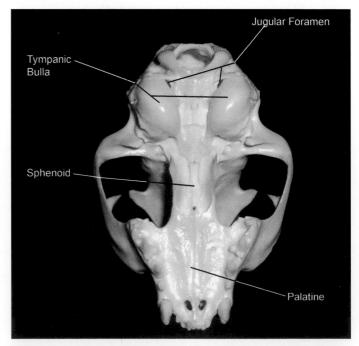

Figure 3.14   Bones of the skull. The mental foramen is an opening through which passes blood vessels and nerve fibers.

Figure 3.16   The ventral skull. The large opening just caudal to the jugular foramen is the foramen magnum, through which the spinal cord passes.

The bone that is deep to the soft tissue that forms the roof of the mouth is the palatine bone. It too is composed of two bones that meet at the midline during fetal development. If these bones do not meet, the animal is born with a gap in the roof of the mouth, and milk or other ingested material can travel up into the nasal cavity and out the nose. This gap is referred to as a cleft palate and can usually be remediated surgically.

The dorsal-most part of the cranium is referred to as the parietal bone. It is considered to be paired in that one plate on each side comes together to form a fixed joint called a suture. Ventral and lateral to the parietal bone is the temporal bone. Caudal to the parietal bone is the occipital bone, and rostral to it is the frontal bone.

On the rostrum are the zygomatic arch, the nasal bone, and incisive bones, as well as the lacrimal bones. The zygomatic arch is the bone ventral to the eye socket, or orbit; in humans, it is called the cheekbone. Technically, the zygomatic arch is made from the zygomatic bone (which forms the rostral part of the arch) and a part of the temporal bone projecting to become its caudal section. The nasal bone consists of the small bones to either side of the nasal passage. The lacrimal bones are small bones forming the ventromedial surface of the orbit. All of these bones are paired. The nasal septum is the wall that divides the nasal passages into right and left. The bone at the caudal nasal passages is called the ethmoid bone. It forms the rostral wall of the skull.

Note that the rostral part of the septum is cartilage, and only the caudal part is composed of bone. It is for this reason that a nose will appear incomplete on looking at a skull. The cartilaginous part does not survive the process of preserving the bone. The lateral orbit in dogs and cats also is not completely bony. There is a small area, which appears as a gap in the preserved skull, where in the living animal there is a ligament. This is in contrast to equines, which do have a completely bony orbit.

The temporal bone has a feature of interest called the bulla. It is a cuplike ventral projection that forms the middle part of the ear. It should be full of air, with the exception of three tiny bones called ossicles, which are an important part of the process of hearing. The ossicles are the smallest bones in the body of dogs and cats (and humans). The opening into the bulla is the medial border of the external auditory canal. As with the nasal septum, the ear canal is mainly cartilaginous. The ear canal is composed of bone only in its medial portion; the area from its entrance is composed of cartilage.

On the ventral surface of the cranium is the palatine bone, which forms the upper border of the oral cavity (the "hard palate"). Cleft palate is the condition mentioned earlier where the two plates that form this bone do not meet. This is a condition that can be genetic or caused by abnormal growth prior to birth. It can cause severe problems with eating and breathing.

The choanae, openings important to the pathway of air through the respiratory tract from the nose and into the throat (pharynx), are on the ventral surface of the skull. The sphenoid is another bone in that area, important in supporting the braincase.

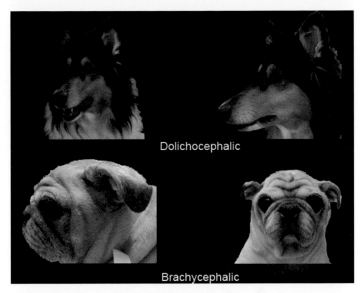

Figure 3.17   The shape of the skull has an effect on everything from how the animal's teeth look to how he or she breathes; a brachycephalic dog has a much shorter nasal passage and oral cavity and can have respiratory problems severe enough to require surgical correction of those structures.

A caudal view of the skull reveals the occipital bone. Here there are two fossae, one on either side of a large opening known as the foramen magnum. These are the occipital fossae. Bony projections in this area are the occipital condyles, an important site for muscle attachment. Slightly rostral to this there are two prominences known as the jugular processes, which frame the area where the jugular veins exit (see Figure 3.16). The foramen magnum accommodates the spinal cord, the nerve fibers that have gathered to bring information to and from the brain.

It will be noticed that certain breeds of dogs and cats have a "flat" appearance to the face. These animals are referred to as brachycephalic (referring to the arch from which the planes of the face form during fetal development) (see Figure 3.17). Distinguishing between brachycephalic, a head shape, and brachiocephalicus, a muscle, will help greatly in terms of increased clarity in describing the patient. Bulldogs and Persian cats are brachycephalic. As a result of the short nasal and oral cavities, among other things, these animals are at greater risk for respiratory problems when under sedation, and special measures are usually undertaken to afford them more oxygen.

On the other hand, a cat or dog with a very long muzzle is said to be dolichocephalic. The Siamese cat and Doberman Pinscher are good examples of these animals. Animals with a medium length of the snout are referred to as mesaticephalic; this includes the tabby cat and the beagle.

Other flat bones

The ribs are a series of flat bones that attach to the spinal column and descend ventrally. The distal part of the rib is composed of cartilage. In the animal with a normal body condition, the ribs should not be easily visible but should be readily palpable. The metacarpal (front paw) and metatarsal (rear paw) bones are considered flat bones by some and short bones by others.

Irregular bones

Of the irregular bones, the best known are the vertebrae, which make up the spinal column (see Figures 3.18 and 3.19). Note that the word spine can refer to a number of things: a feature of some vertebrae, the long thick bundle of nerves known as the spinal cord, or the series of vertebrae that make up the spinal column. When referring to the chain of vertebrae, spinal column is the most correct term.

The vertebrae are divided into five main sections: the cervical, thoracic, lumbar, sacral, and caudal. In cats and dogs, there are 7 cervical (neck), 12 or 13 thoracic (thorax and just distal to the diaphragm), 7 lumbar (caudal dorsum), 3 sacral (intrapelvic), and a variable number of caudal vertebrae. The latter are the ones that make up the tail. (A good piece of trivia is that the giraffe has the same number of cervical vertebrae as the dog. In fact, all mammals except the manatee and her relatives have seven cervical vertebrae.)

The vertebrae are known only by capital letter and number with three exceptions, which have actual names. The cranial-most vertebra is known as the atlas (named for the mythical man who held up the world, just as the atlas helps support the skull). The bone directly caudal to it is the axis. The other named vertebra, the anticlinal vertebra, will be discussed in a moment. Other vertebrae are labeled by their section of the vertebral column and their position along the chain. For example, the atlas

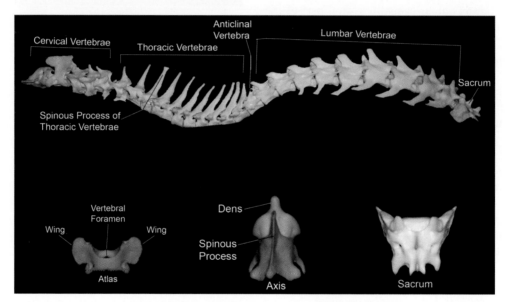

Figure 3.18   At the top is a picture of the complete vertebral column (spinal column) from the lateral view. Below it are photographs of three important vertebrae: the atlas and axis (the first two cervical vertebrae, in that order) and the sacrum, which is three fused vertebrae in dogs and cats and is the point from which the caudal vertebrae depend.

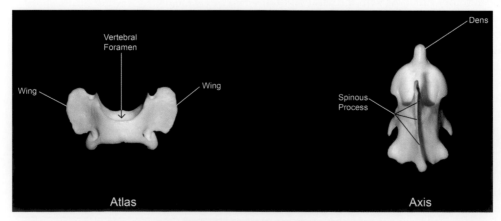

Figure 3.19   The atlas is the cranial-most of the vertebrae, followed by the axis. One way to remember it is that, just as "t" comes before "x," the atlas comes before the axis. Note the dens, which is congenitally absent in some dogs.

is also known as C1, indicating that it is the first cervical vertebra. A radiographic report may indicate that there is a fracture at T3, meaning the third thoracic vertebra.

There are a number of features of vertebrae. The atlas has two lateral projections called the wings. The axis has a small projection that sits in the vertebral foramen of the atlas. This projection is called the dens. Abnormality of this structure (particularly, if it is absent or foreshortened) is associated with neurologically based difficulty with ambulation. The large dorsal projection of the axis is the spinous process of the axis.

The thoracic vertebrae are distinguished by large dorsal projections also called spinous processes. For example, we would discuss the spinous process of the third thoracic vertebra if, for example, there were a fracture or abnormality there. It is in the thoracic spinal column that the anticlinal vertebra is found. It will be noted that the spinous processes of the thoracic vertebrae point caudally, up until the 11th thoracic vertebra (in most dogs and cats). Then a somewhat smaller vertebral spinous process points cranially. It is therefore called the anticlinal vertebra as it inclines in the opposite direction, and it is important because it is a good landmark when looking at radiographs.

The lumbar vertebrae have short spinous processes. They do, however, have long transverse processes, which have the appearance of wings, making them easy to identify.

The sacral vertebrae in dogs and cats are actually fused together and are referred to collectively as the sacrum. There are three bones that have no space between them and a very short vertebral spinous process.

The caudal vertebrae make up the tail of the animal. Most "tail-less" animals actually have at least one or two caudal vertebrae. As dogs and cats have tails of different lengths, there is a variable number of caudal vertebrae in most species and in different breeds of each species.

The sternebrae are irregular bones that run along the ventral surface of the thorax. The cranial-most point of the sternum is called the manubrium, and the caudal-most the xiphoid. This last is an important landmark; most abdominal surgeries, and all ovariohysterectomies ("spays"), have an instruction to prepare the surgical area in some relation to the xiphoid. Note that in primates, the sternum is a single piece of bone.

Equines

There are a few notes about the skeletal features of equines that are important (see Figure 3.20). There is only one digit on each leg. (Ruminants, in contrast, have two on each limb.) It is fascinating that an animal weighing around or even more than 1000 lbs depends on one digit on each leg.

Distal to the carpus or tarsus in each limb is a single metacarpal/metatarsal bone. This is metacarpal/metatarsal bone number 3. There are vestigial remnants of the second and third metacarpal/metatarsals, which are short thin projections on either side of the proximal metacarpal/metatarsal. These are commonly referred to as the "splints," or splint bones.

The distal phalangeal bone, P3, is encased in the hoof and is referred to as the coffin bone. Repeated stress on the limb (or

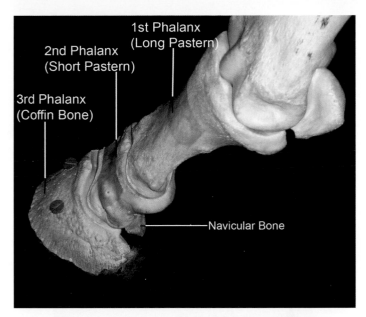

Figure 3.20   The equine lower limb. The caudal-most bone, distal to the navicular, is phalanx 3, also known as the coffin bone. The short bone proximal to it is the short pastern, and the one proximal to it the long pastern. The navicular bone has an important role to play in joint movement.

other causes, such as nutritional issues) can cause laminitis, or inflammation of the layers of the hoof. The swelling can be associated with a change in the angle of the coffin bone to the point where it actually tilts straight down. Basically, the horse is standing on the point of the "toe." As might be imagined, this is extremely painful and can be very difficult to treat.

In the horse, a particularly important sesamoid bone is the navicular bone, which sits just caudally to P3. It serves an important function in relation to tendons and ligaments in the area. As such, it can cause severe problems if the area is inflamed.

Bovines

In contrast to equines, each bovine limb has two digits (see Figure 3.21). The space between the digits is known as the interdigital cleft. In the living animal, there is a cutaneous gland that produces a pheromone in that area.

The bone that isn't

In humans, the clavicle is a bone that connects the sternum to the scapula. In cats, the clavicle is vestigial, a small, thin, sticklike structure that serves no particular purpose. It is important to know about, as it might appear to be a bone chip when viewing a radiograph. Note that there are species, such as rabbits and rodents, that do have a clavicle.

Bird bones

Avians have a special bone structure (see Figure 3.22). Unlike the popular conception, bird bones are not hollow. However,

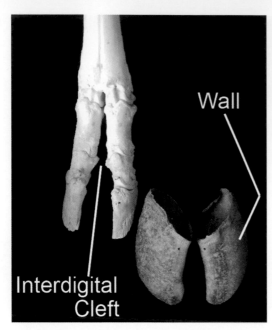

Figure 3.21 The bovine limb has two digits, each with the same three phalangeal bones as the dog and cat. The hoof is also in two parts, joined at the interdigital cleft. The wall of the hoof is indicated.

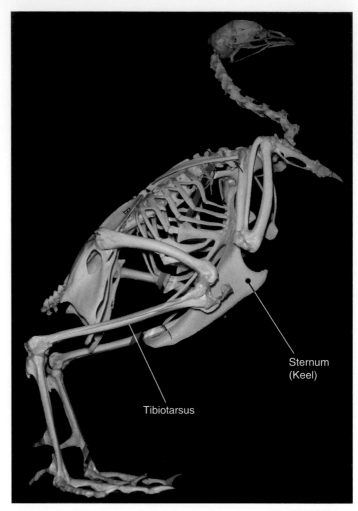

Figure 3.22 The skeleton of the bird. The tibiotarsus is a fused "joint." Note the large sternum ("keel"), perfect for attachment of the powerful pectoral muscles needed for flight.

they are pneumatized (except for the skull); that is, they have many hollowed-out areas, like the recesses of a sponge. This decreases the overall weight of the animal, assisting its ability to fly. Some of the concave areas are connected to the air sacs, which do the job of pulling air into the body. As a result of this, bone fractures can also cause respiratory complications.

There are other differences between avians, and dogs and cats. For example, the avian tibia and tarsus are fused. There are varying numbers of digits per limb, depending on the breed, but the digits of the thoracic limb do not bear any weight. The thoracic limbs of the bird are the bony component of the wings. They still have a humerus, radius, and ulna, although the size and shape of the bones differ a great deal in the various breeds. The sternum, also known as the keel for its resemblance to that part of a boat, is a large, single bone that is very prominent, reinforcing its importance as the anchor for the major muscles of flight.

Review questions

1 Give an example of a flat bone.
2 What is the proper name of the shaft of a long bone?
3 How many phalangeal bones are there in each digit?
4 What is the name of the cranial-most vertebra?
5 What type of bone is the patella?

Clinical case resolution: Newborn puppy

Examination of the puppy's oral cavity revealed that the plates of the palatal bones never came together to form a single palatine bone. The space between them allows food to travel up into the nasal cavity. Food can thus either come out of the nose or up into the airway, causing coughing or sneezing. This can cause food to be aspirated into the lungs, which can cause severe respiratory disease. This problem was readily fixed surgically, and the puppy developed normally thereafter.

Chapter **4** Muscle Anatomy

Clinical case: Cat with epaxial muscle atrophy

A cat is brought into the clinic because she is not as active as usual and has not been eating well. The doctor makes a note in the chart that there is "epaxial muscle atrophy."

The study of muscles and muscle groups is crucial to the understanding of normal and abnormal function not just in relation to ambulation but also to identifying or at least suspecting other disease states. The example above is not a muscle disease itself but a symptom of another problem. This will become clear by the end of the chapter.

Introduction

This section will introduce the various muscles and muscle groups that make up the bulk of the mammalian body. The reader is encouraged to use some of the online resources that accompany this text to help the visualization of these structures. Appendix 3 contains specific information about some of the muscle insertions and origins.

Please refer to Appendix 1, which gives some tips on dissection. When dissecting out muscle, it is useful to remove the white, spiderweb-like material that surrounds it. It is a type of connective tissue, which should be removed in order to see the muscle clearly. It can be brushed away fairly easily. The very tough, flat, white, or silver connective tissue that encases some muscles or muscle connections is known as muscle fascia. It is generally stuck to the muscle tissue closely; if it is necessary to remove it to see beneath it, use blunt dissection to avoid cutting into the muscle below. A large area of fascia covers the muscles on the dorsum in the area of the lumbar spinal column. This is known as the thoracolumbar fascia.

There are three main types of muscle: cardiac, skeletal, and smooth. Cardiac muscle is often put into a separate category because the heart muscle has some components that look like skeletal muscle and some like smooth muscle. As will be discussed in the physiology section, smooth muscles usually function without the animal having to consciously think about

Anatomy and Physiology for Veterinary Technicians and Nurses: A Clinical Approach, First Edition. Robin Sturtz and Lori Asprea.
© 2012 John Wiley & Sons, Inc. Published 2012 by John Wiley & Sons, Inc.

moving them. The heart too moves in this fashion, but its structure has enough skeletal characteristics that a compromise category was created.

Skeletal muscle

Skeletal muscle does the major work of locomotion and strength maneuvers. There are four skeletal muscle shapes. They are strap, pennate, spindle, and sphincter.

All skeletal muscles have "stripes" or striations along their surface, making them stand out from smooth muscle tissue. Skeletal muscle is often referred to as striated muscle. A pennate muscle is one that is shaped like an elongated oval with horizontal or oblique striations. A strap muscle is one that forms a long, thin rectangle. Spindle muscles have fibers that run longitudinally and are shaped like a pennate muscle. A sphincter muscle has a series of circular layers around a central opening. Note that there are also some sphincters made of smooth muscle, such as that of the anal sphincter.

Skeletal muscle is composed of fibers, each of which is a single cell. Bundles of fibers are called fasciculi (single, fasciculus). The fasciculi are attached to each other by connective tissue. The entire group of fasciculi is covered by a connective tissue sheath called the epimysium, which is the part immediately seen when looking at the muscle during dissection (see Figure 4.1). The part the epimysium encircles is referred to as the belly of the muscle. The belly is known as a "head" when there is more than one next to each other and working together. For example, the biceps muscle is composed of two heads, or muscle bellies, which function as a unit.

The origin of any muscle or muscle group is defined as the proximal-most, cranial-most, or central-most connection of a muscle or tendon to the body, and the insertion is the connection distal-most, caudal-most, or furthest away from the median plane of the body. There are some exceptions to this, which we will discuss below. In most cases, the origin is the more fixed point of the muscle, and the insertion the area where the greatest movement occurs.

The various connective tissue sheets converge at either end of many skeletal muscles to form tendons. They are dense, regular fibrous tissue. Tendons are composed mostly of collagen, a tough protein. They are present at the insertion and origin of the muscle. Tendons usually connect to bone. Some tendons are short and flat; others are long and thin. Sometimes, one muscle connects directly to another by way of fibrous material that is not formed as a tendon. This connection is a special type of joint called an aponeurosis. The linea alba ("white line") is the best known of these and will be discussed later; it connects two of the superficial muscles of the abdomen.

Muscles are supplied by arteries, veins, nerve fibers, and lymphatic vessels. The latter runs through the loose connective tissue and fascia surrounding the muscle fibers. Tendons, on the other hand, are poorly vascularized, if at all. Among other things, this means that they do not heal well when injured as the inflammatory cells of the blood cannot reach them.

We can characterize skeletal muscles as either superficial or deep. We will take a regional approach to the study of the anatomy, starting with the head. In each case, we will describe the superficial muscles first and then work to the deeper layers. Once the superficial muscles of each area are identified, transect these muscles through their middle to reveal the layer underneath (i.e., cut them in half at the center so that they can be opened like the leaves of a book). In this manner, one can fold back and reestablish each layer for later study. In preserved organic materials, muscle will usually appear pink or gray. In the living animal, they are a red or brick color. The following muscles are skeletal, unless otherwise noted.

The head and neck

The superficial layer of muscle on the head is called the platysma (see Figure 4.2). It is a very thin layer and can be difficult to

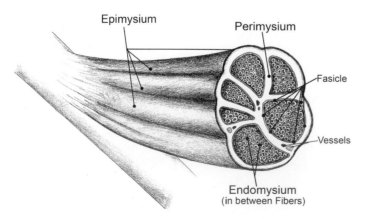

Figure 4.1   The structure of a muscle fascicle.

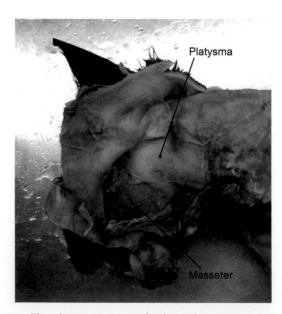

Figure 4.2   The platysma is a superficial muscle encompassing most of the head. The masseter, one of the powerful muscles of chewing, is deep to it.

separate from the dermis. Running from the zygomatic arch to the mandible is the masseter muscle. This is a massive muscle which is crucial to chewing and moving the jaw. Running from the parietal and frontal bones to the mandible is the temporalis muscle. It lies somewhat dorsal to the masseter. Certain neurological diseases can cause the lateral surfaces of the head to have a concave appearance, caused by the atrophy of the temporalis (e.g., myasthenia gravis, a rare neuromuscular disease in dogs).

The orbicularis oculi are muscle fibers that surround the eye, and orbicularis oris are those surrounding the mouth. Digastricus is a large muscle forming the floor of the oral cavity, important in opening the mouth. The tongue is a large muscle composed of several sections. The muscles of the tongue are the styloglossus, genioglossus, and hyoglossus. They function as one muscle. The buccinator on each side runs from the maxilla to the mandible and is equivalent to the interior oral ("cheek") muscle.

The preauricular muscles are those rostral to the pinna and assist in moving the pinna to pinpoint sounds in various locations. In mammals that depend to a great extent on hearing in lieu of poor eyesight (bats, rabbits), these muscles are crucial to survival.

The superficial muscles of the neck include the brachiocephalicus (literally, "arm head"; the root word "ceph" refers to the head), which runs from the mastoid process of the temporal bone toward the scapula. Another superficial muscle of the neck is the sternocephalicus, which runs to the sternum from the mastoid bone. Trapezius goes from the neck to the thoracic vertebrae, running along the dorsal and lateral surface of the thorax.

Deeper muscles that run along the ventral neck include sternocephalicus and sternothyroideus. These are strap muscles. They run along or are ventral to the trachea. They are important landmarks in doing a tracheotomy as they must be pushed aside in order to visualize the trachea.

The thorax

There are scattered areas of muscle tissue around the subcutaneous layer of the skin along the thorax and abdomen. They have fascicles running in a cranial-caudal direction. They are involved in the fasciculation ("twitching") of the skin, which dogs and cats engage in when they are stimulated. The particular muscles involved in this movement are called the panniculus muscles.

Superficial muscles of the thorax include the superficial and deep pectorals (see Figure 4.3). The name deep pectoral is misleading as it is in fact a superficial muscle. The pectorals are present on the ventral thorax and run from the sternum to the proximal thoracic limb. The superficial pectoral is cranial to the deep pectoral. Both have some fibers that run in a "V" shape. In the dog and cat, these muscles are rather thin. In avians, the pectorals are an important part to the ability to fly and are very thick and powerful.

For the rest of this chapter, refer to Figures 4.4–4.14. We will keep muscle groups together in discussion. To see where they actually appear on the body, follow the labels on the photographs.

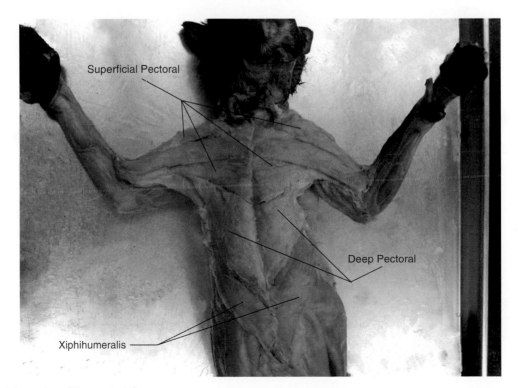

Figure 4.3   Superficial muscles of the ventral thorax.

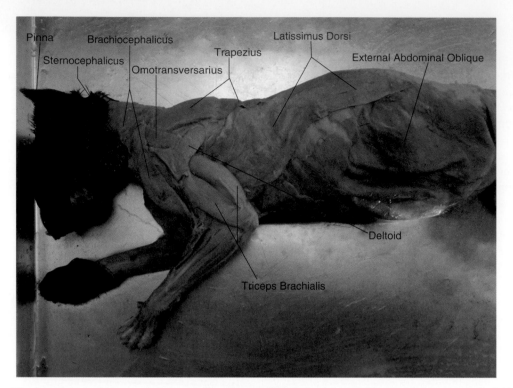

Figure 4.4 Muscles of the lateral neck, thorax, and abdomen. The pinna is the outermost part of the ear; it is composed of skin-covered cartilage but does have musculature surrounding it, allowing it to turn and capture sound.

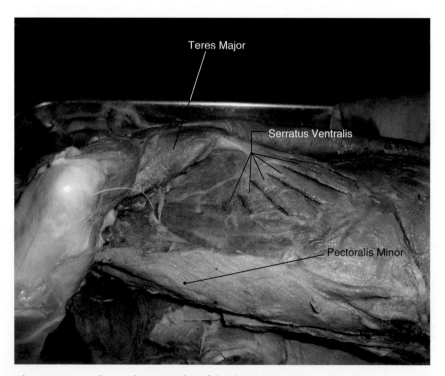

Figure 4.5 The teres major and serratus ventralis are deep muscles of the thorax. Note that pectoralis minor is another way of saying deep pectoral. The head is to the left.

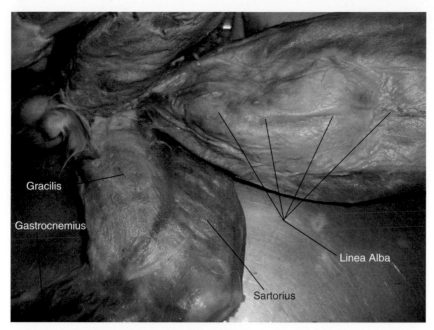

Figure 4.6 Muscles of the lower ventrum and medial thigh. The linea alba is an aponeurosis (a fibrous connection between muscles) and is an important surgical landmark. The head is to the right.

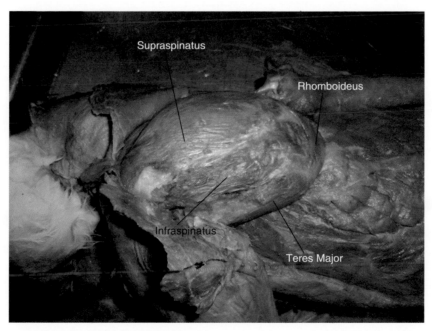

Figure 4.7 Muscles on and around the scapula. The head is to the left.

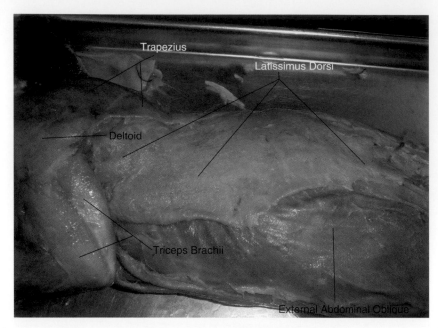

Figure 4.8   Muscles along the thoracic limb, dorsum, and lateral abdomen. The head is to the left.

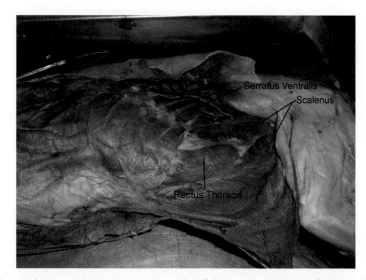

Figure 4.9   The cat is in left lateral recumbency, with the head to the right of the picture. The superficial muscles have been reflected (bent aside) to afford a better view.

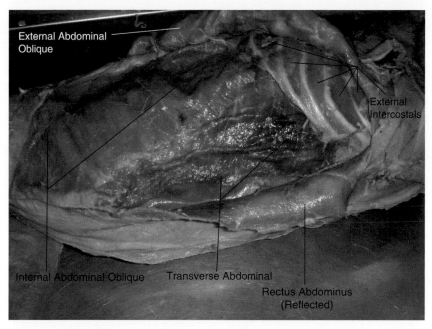

Figure 4.10   Deep muscles of the thorax and abdomen. The head is to the right.

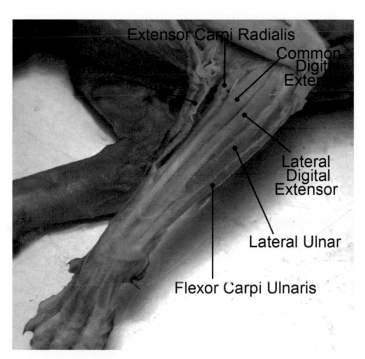

Figure 4.11   Muscles of the antebrachium. The caudal muscles are mostly flexors. The craniolateral muscles are mostly extensors. The exception is the lateral ulnar muscle, which is a flexor.

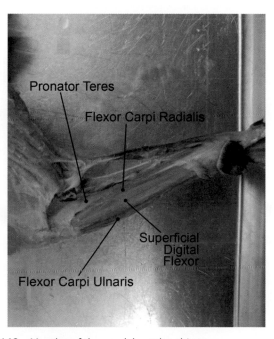

Figure 4.12   Muscles of the caudal antebrachium.

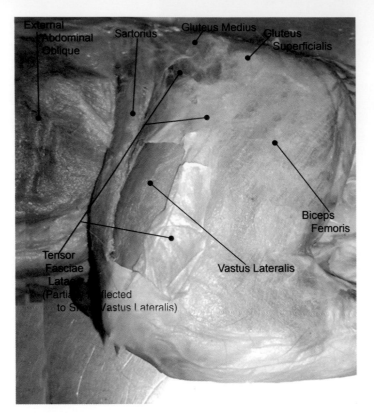

Figure 4.13   Muscles of the lateral dorsum and lateral pelvic limb.

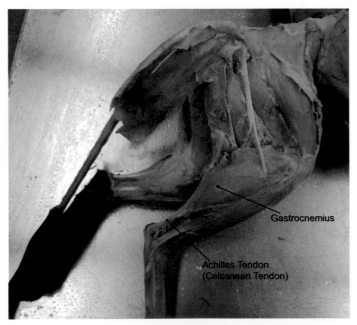

Figure 4.14   Muscles of the pelvic limb.

Another superficial muscle is the deltoid, which runs from the spine of the scapula to the deltoid tuberosity of the humerus. The latissimus dorsi runs from the thoracolumbar spine to the humerus. It is one of the rare muscles where the origin is caudal to the insertion. It is a large but thin muscle and needs to be carefully pulled away from the trunk in order to observe the muscles deep to it; use blunt dissection to separate it rather than a scalpel.

The serratus muscle is actually a series of sections. The largest parts are the serratus dorsalis and the serratus ventralis. Dorsalis rides along the dorsum of the thorax and ventralis along the lateral surface. Ventralis is just deep to the latissimus dorsi. The lateral section of the serratus ventralis is arranged in bands of tissue that form flat sections running at an angle, appearing much like the bars of a marimba. It is from this "serrated" appearance that the muscle draws its name. This muscle helps to form the sling that holds the scapula to the body wall.

Deeper muscles of the thorax include the supraspinatus and the infraspinatus, thick muscles that fill the fossae on either lateral surface of the spine of the scapula. Other muscles of the deep thorax include the internal and external intercostals, which are deep to the serratus ventralis and are important in breathing. The externals are superficial to the internals. Lastly, there is the scalenus muscle, which extends from the dorsal neck of the animal to the cervical vertebrae. Scalenus is also involved in respiration.

A term that has some clinical significance is "thoracic girdle." The term girdle implies encircling the body. The thoracic girdle includes the latissimus dorsi, trapezius, serratus ventralis, and the pectoral muscles. They are all involved in connecting the thoracic limb to the trunk and function as a joint during movements such as shifting weight from one leg to the other. These muscles are the only things that attach the thoracic limb to the body as there are no bony attachments. In contrast to the thoracic girdle, the pelvic girdle refers to bone only; that is, the pelvic limbs are connected to the rest of the skeleton by a direct joint between the femur and the pelvis.

Muscles associated with the shoulder include the omotransversarius, originating at the wing of the atlas and going to the spine of the scapula, and the rhomboideus. The rhomboideus is deep to trapezius and runs from the skull and neck to the scapula. The trapezius is part of this group as well.

The dorsum

Some muscles of the dorsum deserve special mention. The group of muscles known as epaxial muscles run dorsally to the transverse processes of some of the vertebrae, including particularly the lumbar vertebrae. This group includes the muscles iliocostal, longissimus (which has four sections), and transversospinalis. These muscles are important because they assist in respiration. They are often the site of intramuscular injections. They must be handled gently in conducting any kind of spinal surgery, such as laminectomy. They are particularly sensitive to significant weight loss and will show mild atrophy early in the process of losing weight. This atrophy will be particularly noticeable if the weight loss is long-standing or dramatic. As such, these muscles give a good informal clue as to the state of health of the animal. They lie just underneath the epaxial aponeurosis.

The hypaxial muscles are deep to the epaxials. They include the major psoas and minor psoas and the iliacus. They help flex the spinal column and move the pelvic limbs. Due to their location, they are also referred to as sublumbar muscles.

The abdomen

Superficial muscles of the abdomen include the internal and external abdominal oblique muscles. Their fibers are oriented at an angle to each other, with the striations flowing in opposite directions. They are found on the ventral and lateral abdomen. They meet at the ventral abdominal midline at the linea alba, a thick fibrous line described above as an aponeurosis. The linea alba is a convenient place to make an incision when doing abdominal surgery, if for no other reason than that it is easy to see and allows the surgeon to avoid cutting into the muscle of the body wall. Ovariohysterectomies (spays) are always begun at the linea alba in dogs and cats. The internal abdominal oblique at its caudal-most part becomes the cremaster muscle in males. This muscle plays an important part in reproductive activities.

Deeper abdominal muscles include the rectus abdominus, running cranially to caudally down the center of the abdomen, and the transverse abdominal, which follows a course from one lateral surface to the other. The rectus abdominus is covered by a sheath, which can be used to place sutures to anchor the skin and body wall during abdominal surgery.

The pelvis

The medial and superficial gluteal muscles run from the pelvis to the femur. The medial gluteal muscle is actually cranial to the superficial gluteal muscle. There is a deep gluteal muscle as well. Interestingly, despite its sizable rump, the ruminant does not have a superficial gluteal muscle.

Other muscles of the pelvis include the internal and external obturators, which cover the obturator foramen. The gemelli (from the Greek word for twins) help connect the pelvis and the femur as does the quadratus femoris.

The perineum refers to the area under the tail and lateral to the anus. It also includes the anus. The anus itself actually has two sphincter muscles—an external sphincter and an internal sphincter. The external anal sphincter is composed of skeletal muscle and is a voluntary muscle. The reason that Fluffy can wait until the proper time and place to defecate relates to the control this muscle provides. The internal anal sphincter is composed of the smooth or involuntary muscle, which is why the animal sometimes cannot hold out if the urge is strong enough.

The coccygeus is a muscle that goes from the ischium to the tail. The levator ani also goes from the pelvis to the perineum. It slings around the rectum and is important in the process of defecation. In any surgery involving the anus or the anal glands, it is crucial not to sever this muscle. If it is disrupted, the animal may become incontinent.

The limbs

We now come to a discussion of the limbs. Muscles of the limbs are often described as extrinsic or intrinsic. Extrinsic muscles are those that connect the limb to the body. Intrinsic muscles have both their origin and their insertion on the limb itself.

The thoracic limb

Extrinsic muscles of the thoracic limb include the brachiocephalicus, trapezius, omotransversarius, latissimus dorsi, deltoid, and superficial pectoral. Triceps brachii and biceps brachii originate on the scapula and insert on the olecranon or radius, respectively. The tendon of origin of the biceps brachii is important in flexing the shoulder. As mentioned, the scapula is considered to be a part of the thoracic limb in that the scapula does not have any bony attachment to the rest of the skeleton. Teres major and teres minor are deep muscles involved in the flexion of the shoulder joint.

Deeper muscles of the brachium include brachialis and anconeus. These muscles are involved in flexion and extension of the elbow, respectively.

The muscles of the dorsolateral antebrachium are almost all involved in extension of the limb, particularly relating to the paw and digits. Going clockwise toward the lateral surface, these muscles include the extensor carpi radialis, common digital extensor, lateral digital extensor, and lateral ulnar. The supinator muscle is deep to these. The only flexor muscle in this group is the lateral ulnar.

The caudal surface of the antebrachium includes the flexor carpi radialis, the flexor carpi ulnaris (which has two heads), and the superficial digital flexor. The deeper muscles include the deep digital flexor, pronator teres, and pronator quadratus. The deep digital flexor has three heads. All of these muscles are flexors. Reference to the interosseous "muscle" actually indicates ligaments that run from the metacarpals to the digits. In horses, they form a thick bundle called the suspensory ligament, which is important in the stay apparatus.

The stay apparatus is a vital part of locomotion in horses and cows. Actually, the stay apparatus has to do with the animal at rest. The large amount of weight that these large animals put on their relatively thin legs would ordinarily cause significant fatigue and possibly injury. In order to give the muscles and joints of the limb time to rest, the ligaments, tendons, and muscles are constructed in such a way that weight is distributed over three limbs at any one time in the standing animal. The "free" limb does not bear weight and usually remains in a flexed position with the tip of the hoof on the ground. Periodically, the animal will shift his weight to give another limb a rest. The result is that the wear and tear on the limbs is considerably less. The combination of muscles, ligaments, and tendons that allow this shifting of weight is called the stay apparatus.

Carnivores, some omnivores, and pigs are the only animals that can supinate (turn the palmar/plantar surface upward) and pronate (the reverse of supinate) the distal extremity. Herbivores generally cannot. The latter do not have the pronator muscles, and their radius and ulna are fused.

The pelvic limb

The muscles of the pelvic limb are generally quite large and very powerful. Most mammals use the pelvic limbs to accelerate movement, while the muscles of the thoracic limbs are more involved in supporting the heavier structure of the head.

The middle, deep, and superficial gluteals all connect the pelvis and the proximal thigh and are found on the dorsolateral surface of the limb. Lateral muscles of the pelvic limb include the biceps femoris, a very large muscle running all the way from the pelvis to the tarsus. The tensor fasciae latae runs from the pelvis to the stifle. However, only the proximal section of it looks like muscle; the rest of it is composed of fascia, which has a silvery appearance. To see the deeper muscles, cut through the fascia, not the proximal part of the muscle. Semitendinosis is a muscle of the lateral and caudal surface of the limb. It is not recommended to use this muscle for injection as it is just superficial and caudal to the ischiatic (sciatic) nerve. If an injection is made into this muscle, and the sciatic nerve is punctured, it might render the limb useless. The risk is significantly greater with smaller dogs and cats as the distance to the nerve is even shorter. (We generally use the cranial side of the limb, such as the cranial portion of the sartorius muscle.) Deep to the biceps femoris muscle is the vastus lateralis. As the name implies, it too is a large, powerful muscle.

The medial thigh includes muscles such as gracilis and sartorius, with the former medial to the latter. These muscles extend to the stifle. Sartorius has two heads in dogs, one in cats. Semimembranosis extends from the ischiatic tuberosity to the femur and the tibia by way of two heads. The muscle runs medial to semitendinosis and wraps around the cranial section of the proximal thigh. The cranial portion of this muscle is often used for injection, particularly in cats. (On occasion, the epaxial muscles are used for this purpose as well.)

The quadriceps muscle runs both superficially and deeply in the thigh by way of its four heads. All four join to form one very thick tendon that inserts onto the tibial tuberosity. The tendon of insertion of the quadriceps is also called the patellar tendon. Contained within it is the patella itself. In horses and ruminants, there are three patellar ligaments associated with this tendon. The ability of the animal to use them to stabilize the patella in one position or another is another important part of the stay apparatus.

The crus (the area from the stifle to the tarsus) contains the long and lateral digital extensors on its cranial surface and the gastrocnemius muscle on the caudal surface. The cranial tibial muscle is a superficial muscle of the cranial crus. The gastrocnemius has two bellies and is the equivalent to the human calf muscle. The tendon of insertion of the gastrocnemius muscle ends at the calcaneus and is thus known as the calcanean tendon. It is the equivalent to the human Achilles tendon and is extremely thick (Figure 4.14).

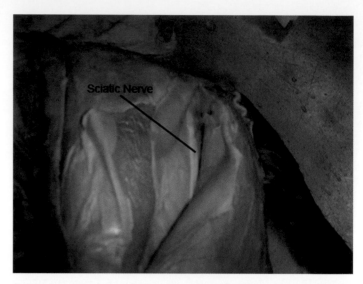

Figure 4.15   The biceps femoris is reflected for better viewing. The white spaghetti-like structure that is seen coursing distally into the proximal gastrocnemius is the sciatic (ischiatic) nerve.

The crus of the mammal also has a deep digital flexor and superficial digital flexor muscle, both involved in flexion of the digits and extension of the tarsus. The soleus muscle is found in cats but not in dogs, and extends along the caudal crus to join the lateral head of the gastrocnemius.

Smooth muscle

This chapter has not yet dealt with the subject of the smooth muscles. These form the walls of some internal organs and vessels. They are mostly triggered by the autonomic nervous system and will be discussed in conjunction with it. In general, smooth muscle does not appear to have the striations of skeletal muscle. While smooth muscle can contract strongly, it is slower to contract than many skeletal muscles.

> ### Clinical case resolution: Cat with epaxial muscle atrophy
>
> *Looking closely at the cat mentioned above, it is easy to see the spinous processes of the thoracic and lumbar vertebrae. They are not surrounded by their usual epaxial muscle tissue, and their outline is readily visible. This is what is meant by epaxial muscle atrophy. Lack of protein will cause muscles to atrophy or "shrink"; a common cause of hypoproteinemia is anorexia. This process does not happen overnight. Thus, seeing epaxial muscle wasting tells the examiner that the animal has not eaten much, if anything, for quite some time. This helps define the time frame for the animal's illness and aids in making a diagnosis. This should always be checked in doing a physical examination on any mammal.*

Review questions

1 List the four types of skeletal muscle.
2 What is the primary difference between smooth muscle and skeletal muscle?
3 Name two superficial muscles of the ventral thorax.
4 What is different about the origin and insertion of the latissimus dorsi, compared to other muscles of the trunk?
5 Name two superficial muscles of the ventral abdomen.
6 Name two muscles of the caudal femoral area. Why do we need to be able to identify them?
7 What is the proper name for the part of the pelvic limb between the stifle and the tarsus? Name two muscles found in that area.
8 Is the extensor carpi radialis on the dorsal or caudal surface of the antebrachium?
9 Name an intrinsic muscle of the scapula.
10 Name an extrinsic muscle of the scapula.
11 What is the linea alba?
12 Where can the muscle "serratus ventralis" be found?

Chapter 5 The Anatomy of Joints

Clinical case: Yorkshire terrier with lameness

A Yorkshire terrier is brought into the clinic by his worried family. He has been holding his right pelvic limb up in the air and cries when someone tries to touch the leg. Occasionally, he will put it down and walk normally, but he then returns to lameness.

Introduction

The study of joints is called arthrology. Joints are junctions between distinct bones or other tissue. They are an articulation, a point where things intersect. In the limbs, these connections allow certain types of movement. In other parts of the body, a joint may be a remnant of an embryonic structure or may delineate a border.

Types of joints

The major types of joints are fibrous, cartilaginous, and synovial.

A fibrous joint represents an area where the borders of bones have met and are connected by way of fibrous (proteinaceous) material. Fibrous joints are generally not mobile, although there are some exceptions. The best-known fibrous joints are the sutures of the skull. These thin areas where the skull bones approach each other during fetal development are somewhat mobile immediately after birth. They continue to ossify and become a solid line. The sutures usually become immobile connections within a short time.

A fontanel is the gap between bones of the skull (usually, the parietal and frontal bones) where the suture is unformed or incomplete. In hydrocephaly (from the root words meaning "water-head"), where excess fluid is produced within the skull, the fontanel may bulge because of the increased fluid pressure. This is often associated with a domed appearance to the skull and is very common in Chihuahuas.

Anatomy and Physiology for Veterinary Technicians and Nurses: A Clinical Approach, First Edition. Robin Sturtz and Lori Asprea.
© 2012 John Wiley & Sons, Inc. Published 2012 by John Wiley & Sons, Inc.

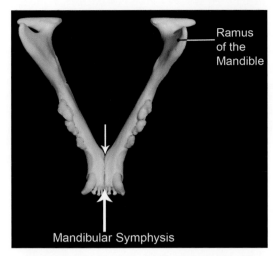

Figure 5.1   The mandibular symphysis is a fibrous joint. A similar joint is present at the medial pubic bone and is referred to as the pubic symphysis.

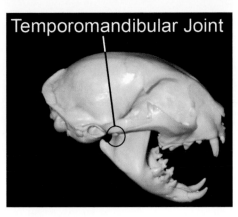

Figure 5.2   The temporomandibular joint is a synovial joint, with one cartilaginous meniscus (disk).

Other fibrous joints include the equine metacarpus and the gomphosis. The gomphosis is the type of fibrous connection found anchoring a tooth to its socket. Loosening this joint when performing a manual tooth extraction is an important part of successful dentistry.

Cartilaginous joints are, as the name implies, connections between bones that are composed of cartilage. The best-known cartilaginous joints are those between the vertebrae. The vertebrae are connected to each other by pads of cartilage called intervertebral disks (IVDs). These connections are considered to be joints in that there is some flexibility along the spinal column, and that movement is facilitated by the IVDs.

The hyoid apparatus is a "U"-shaped series of small bones connecting the temporal bone and the larynx. Most of the joints of this structure are cartilaginous.

There is also a type of joint called fibrocartilaginous, which contains tissue of both types. An example of a fibrocartilaginous joint is the mandibular symphysis (see Figure 5.1). A symphysis is a connection between bones that is firm and is composed of a fibrocartilaginous or cartilaginous material. Symphyses are located along the midline of the structure. They have the appearance of a suture, but the term suture is reserved for the discussion of the skull. The mandibular symphysis is at the most rostral point of the mandible and can be seen as a thin line when looking at the mature skull. It is a location for fracture when severe trauma to the jaw occurs; if the bones of each side of the mandible can shift relative to each other on physical exam, there is most likely an interruption of the mandibular symphysis. Note, however, that in dogs and in ruminants, the mandibular symphysis never completely fuses. There is another large symphysis connecting the two parts of the pubic bone; it is referred to as the pubic symphysis. The slight amount of flexibility in this joint is important to the animal when giving birth. Guinea pigs that are not bred before 6 months of age undergo fusion of the pubic symphysis, making any future farrowing (giving birth) complicated.

Synovial joints

The synovial joint is the one with the most movement. Synovial joints are often contained within a capsule of fibrous material. Lining this capsule (or simply surrounding the joint if no capsule is present) is a connective tissue sheet called synovial membrane. The membrane produces a viscous fluid called synovium. This fluid has the appearance and density of egg white (hence the name, which comes from the Latin word "ovum," meaning egg).

Many synovial joints have one or more menisci. A meniscus is a disk of fibrocartilage that helps to cushion movement within the joint. A ligament is a fibrocartilaginous extension of the joint capsule and adds stability to the joint, as well as preventing the joint from bending too far or in the wrong direction. The temporomandibular joint (TMJ), for example, has a single meniscus (see Figure 5.2).

The bones within the joint capsule are covered at the proximal/distal-most end by a thin layer of cartilage called articular cartilage. The articular cartilage is made of a particular connective tissue called hyaline cartilage. Under normal circumstances, the articular cartilage has a white or light pink color and has the pebbled appearance of ground glass. In older animals, the articular cartilage may appear somewhat yellow. A deep pink or red color, or seeing flakes of material that appear to be scaling off the surface, indicates joint disease.

Some synovial joints include a fibrocartilaginous lip called an articular labrum on the surface of one of the bones. This is particularly found where a concave surface joins with the head of a long bone, such as at either the scapulohumeral or coxofemoral joint. The labrum is somewhat softer than the bone of the fossa, and so it deforms when the bones move against one another to help spread the weight-bearing, as well as allow more synovial fluid to lubricate the joint.

The stifle has a fat pad cranial to the joint capsule. The fat pad deep to the patella leaves a distinct distance between the patella and the distal femur; in cases of disturbance of the ligaments of the stifle, the fat pad will be displaced and will often appear further away on radiography.

Tendons

The thick fibrous material that forms a connection between a muscle and a bone is called a tendon. If that connection reaches over a joint, a great deal of stress is put on the tendon (and thus on the muscle). Some joints have a bursa, which is a sac containing fluid that sits under the tendon, to cushion the movement. In horses, for example, the bursa associated with the shoulder joint is outside of the joint capsule. The bursa actually requires a separate local anesthetic if shoulder surgery is contemplated. In dogs, the tendon of the biceps brachii muscle is covered by a synovial sheath as it travels between the greater and lesser tubercles of the humerus. This sheath is an extension of the capsule of the scapulohumeral joint and reflects the great degree of pressure this tendon sustains.

The skull

The skull has several kinds of joints. The sutures of the skull have been discussed, as has the mandibular symphysis. Within the middle ear (between the tympanic membrane and the cochlea) are three small bones known as the ossicles. The connection between them is ligamentous, but since they allow for slight movement, they may be considered fibrous joints (see Figure 5.3). The ramus of the mandible meets the temporal bone of the skull at a point called the TMJ. This is a synovial joint and has a single meniscus between the ramus and the skull. The TMJ also has a ligament associated with it.

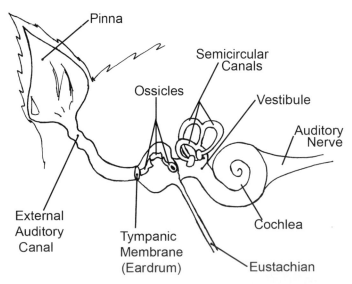

Figure 5.3   The area from the pinna to the tympanic membrane is the outer ear. From the tympanic membrane to the cochlea is the middle ear, housed in the tympanic bulla. This includes the Eustachian tube. The cochlea, semicircular canals, and vestibule form the inner ear; the latter two relate to proprioception.

Note: This drawing is also found in Chapter 17 as it relates to the discussion of the sense of hearing.

The ribs and vertebral column

Moving caudally, the atlantooccipital and the atlantoaxial joints are synovial joints. The former allows dorsoventral movement, and the latter side-to-side movement, of the skull. There are ligaments that help connect the dens to the skull and to the spinal column. The costovertebral joints are "ball-and-socket" synovial joints where the ribs meet the vertebrae. Note that there is another joint distal to this along the rib, the costochondral joint. This is a fibrous joint connecting the bony and the cartilaginous portions of the rib.

The nuchal ligament is a cord-like structure that runs from the cranial spinal column (usually, the axis) to the spinous process of the first thoracic vertebra. It is easily seen in dogs. There is no nuchal ligament in the cat, which may explain the increased flexibility in neck movement in felines. By comparison, there are two nuchal ligaments in the horse and ruminant, most likely reflecting the relatively larger head size. It is discussed in this chapter because, as a ligament, it supports the movement of joints.

The pelvis and hip

The pelvis has several joints. The sacroiliac joint is a relatively immobile joint that connects the sacrum and the ilium. The pubic symphysis was mentioned earlier. Also of note is the sacrotuberous ligament, which runs from the sacrum to the ischiatic tuberosity. It is immobile, and thus not really associated with a joint, but is a stabilizing structure. As with the nuchal ligament, it is present in dogs but not in cats.

The coxofemoral joint is commonly known as the hip. The head of the femur is nested in the acetabulum. This is a synovial joint and has the most range of movement of all the joints involving the limbs. There is a small ligament, the ligament of the femoral head, that helps stabilize the femur within the joint space. An abnormal shape of the head of the femur, and/or a shallow or angled acetabulum, is a cause of lameness. The condition is known as hip dysplasia and is unfortunately common in many dogs, particularly larger breeds.

The shoulder and thoracic limb

The shoulder, or the scapulohumeral joint, involves the intersection of the glenoid fossa of the scapula and the head of the humerus. It is a synovial joint. A congenital condition in some dogs called osteochondrosis often affects the shoulder joint. The elbow (humeroradioulnar) joint involves the condylar intersection with the trochlear notch of the ulna. It too is a synovial joint. There are collateral ligaments (ligaments at the lateral and medial sides of the joint) associated with this joint, preventing excessive lateral movement of the antebrachium relative to the brachium.

The carpus has three sets of joints that are collectively known as the carpal joint. The antebrachiocarpal joint is the proximal-most one, the space between the antebrachium and the proximal carpal bones. The middle carpal joint is that between the proxi-

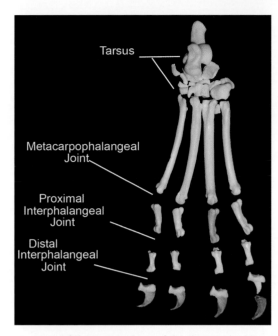

Figure 5.4 Joints of the manus (paw of the thoracic limb). Note that the carpus is actually composed of a number of bones. The same is true for the tarsus. The joint names are the same in pes (paw of the pelvic limb), except that the joint between the metatarsals and the proximal phalanx is the metatarsophalangeal joint.

mal and middle rows of bones. The distal-most of these joints is the carpometacarpal joint. Of the three, this one has the least movement.

The digits have three bones, as we discussed earlier (see Figure 5.4). The joints associated with the digits are the meta-carpophalangeal, proximal interphalangeal, and distal inter-phalangeal. Respectively, these are the joints between the metacarpals and proximal phalangeal bones (P1), the proximal and middle phalangeal bones (P1 and P2), and the middle and distal phalangeal bones (P2 and P3). The interphalangeal joints are synovial joints. Note that in equines, these three joints are commonly known as the fetlock, the long pastern, and the short pastern. There is only one of each phalangeal bone in each leg. The metacarpal/metatarsal bone of consequence is the third; metacarpal/metatarsal bones two and four are also known as the "splint bones." They serve no function and are adhered to metacarpal/metatarsal three.

The pelvic limb

Perhaps the most intricate of the synovial joints in the mammal is the femorotibial joint, commonly known as the stifle. This joint includes a medial and lateral meniscus, a medial and lateral collateral ligament, and is supported by a patellar ligament. The patellar ligament is actually a part of the patellar tendon; the ligament provides further support by connecting the patella and the tibial tuberosity. While the stifle has a major role in weight-

bearing and locomotion in all mammals, the larger animals such as equines and ruminants have a particularly large ratio of body surface to limb surface. This puts even more strain on the stifle. These animals have three patellar ligaments, which assist in weight-bearing.

Two major ligaments of the stifle are the cranial and caudal cruciate ligaments. In dogs, damage to the cranial cruciate is a common cause of stifle-related lameness. The cranial cruciate ligament runs from the caudolateral femur to the cranial tibia. If this ligament does not function correctly, the tibia can slide forward of the femur; testing for this abnormal movement, known as the drawer test, is a part of any canine or feline lameness exam. The caudal cruciate ligament runs from the craniomedial femur to the caudal tibia.

The joints of the tarsus and the distal limb are analogous to those in the thoracic limb. The difference is mostly in the names of the bones, and in the use of the root tarso (as in tarsometatarsal joint).

A note on avians: Birds have somewhat different structures. The tibia and tarsus are fused in many breeds rather than separated by a joint. There is no pubic symphysis, given that the pelvis of the bird is one fused structure. The bones of the skull are also fused in one piece.

Clinical case resolution: Yorkshire terrier with lameness

The dog described at the start of this chapter has a condition known as luxating patella. The patella literally slips out of position and slides to one side of the stifle joint. It is fairly common in small-breed dogs and varies in severity from almost unnoticeable to the inability to bear weight noted above. This dog required surgery, after which he was fine.

Review questions

1 What joint on the canine limb is analogous to the equine fetlock?
2 Name a ligament that dogs have but cats do not have.
3 Name the features of the stifle joint.
4 What are the three major categories of joints?
5 What color should the articular cartilage be?
6 List three synovial joints.
7 What is the difference between a suture and a symphysis?
8 What is an articular labrum? Where would you find one on the dog?
9 What is the drawer test? What part of the joint does it test?
10 What joint is involved in the movement of a dog's head from side to side?

Chapter **6** Anatomy of the Nervous System

Clinical case: Intramuscular injection

In giving a routine intramuscular injection to a dog in the caudal thigh, one usually uses the proximal part of the limb. The technician inserts the needle next to the semitendinosus muscle. The doctor stops her and suggests she use the cranial thigh instead. The reason for this will become clear as we discuss the nervous system.

Introduction

This chapter will cover some of the major anatomical structures associated with the system of nerve fibers running throughout the body of an animal. At the end of this book is a guide (Appendix 2) that provides a mnemonic device for remembering the names of the 12 cranial nerves. Material regarding the function of the nerves will be covered in the nerve physiology chapter.

The neuron

A neuron is a single cell and is also referred to as a nerve fiber (see Figure 6.1). The body of the cell is referred to as a soma. Small fibers that branch from the soma and each other are referred to as dendrites. The long, relatively thick extension from the soma toward another neuron is called an axon. The space between the distal end of the axon and either another neuron or a final receptor is called a synapse. The rounded part of the distal axon is referred to as the terminal bouton (also known as the synaptic bulb). It is from the terminal bouton that neurotransmitters are sent across the synapse to stimulate the next neuron in the sequence. Neurotransmitters are chemicals crucial to neurological function and will also be discussed in Chapter 18.

Nerves in the brain or in the spinal cord are referred to as part of the central nervous system. Other nerves are considered peripheral nerves, meaning that they directly branch from the central nervous system. All nerves do not necessarily end or begin in the brain; peripheral nerves can arise and/or return directly from or to the spinal cord, particularly those nerves involved in reflex or autonomic responses.

Anatomy and Physiology for Veterinary Technicians and Nurses: A Clinical Approach, First Edition. Robin Sturtz and Lori Asprea.
© 2012 John Wiley & Sons, Inc. Published 2012 by John Wiley & Sons, Inc.

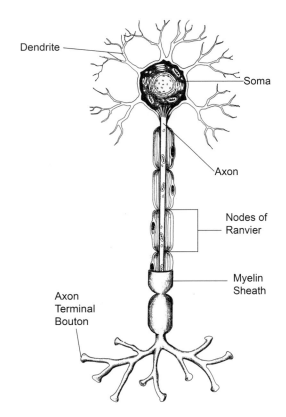

Figure 6.1   The neuron.

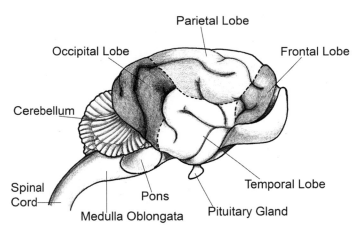

Figure 6.2   Functional sections of the brain.

A bundle of nerve fibers that arise from a common origin in the central nervous system is known as a fasciculus. The major fasciculi have specific names. Not all fasciculi, and certainly not all nerve fibers, have names. Most major nerves derive their names from their location. Some, particularly those associated with the brain stem, are named for their function. When the layperson refers to a nerve, he or she is referring to a fasciculus.

Some basic vocabulary: A collection of nerve cell bodies within the brain is referred to as a nucleus. A "nucleus" that occurs outside the brain is known as a ganglion. Some of these are readily seen on dissection and appear as a small white or beige swelling with a number of nerves radiating out from them. Many ganglia are associated with the autonomic nervous system.

The brain

The brain is covered by a series of layers called meninges. The outermost layer is called the dura mater; it is essentially fused to the skull in most mammalian species, just as the periosteum is fused to the bone. Deep to the dura mater is the subdural space, deep to which is the arachnoid membrane. The space deep to it, the subarachnoid space, is where the cerebrospinal fluid circulates around the brain. The innermost layer, which sits directly on the brain, is called the pia mater.

An expansion of the subarachnoid space, called the cisterna magna, is an area near the transition of the cerebellum into the medulla oblongata. It is from this space that we sample cerebrospinal fluid to check for certain diseases; the common name of this procedure is a cervical or cisternal spinal tap. The animal should be in lateral recumbency, with its nose at a 90° angle to the spinal column; in other words, you should be facing the dorsal neck, with the spinal column as straight as possible, and the space as accessible as possible. Placement of the sampling needle should be on the midline, between the occipital condyles (cranially) and the wings of the atlas (caudally). As might be imagined, serious damage can be inflicted if the needle penetrates the spinal cord, so the animal must be under general anesthesia. Another space for sampling cerebrospinal fluid can also be utilized by sampling from an area between two of the distal lumbar vertebrae; the exact location depends to some extent on the size of the animal.

In the brain, the cell layers on the upper layer of the cerebrum are referred to as gray matter. Deep to that is the white matter, so called because parts of the nerve fibers are covered by a lipid-based insulating material known as myelin, which is whitish in color.

The surface of the mammalian brain is composed of a series of folds (see Figures 6.2 and 6.3). The folds are called gyri (singular: gyrus), and the valleys between them are sulci (sulcus). The gyri help increase the surface area of the brain and allow for more brain function. Avians have a smoother brain surface, which we associate with the capacity for fewer complex or integrative thought processes. Animals without a true brain, such as sea stars, are not believed to have any higher brain function, and presumably do not interpret stimuli, but merely react reflexively.

The lobes of the brain are areas named for their location relative to the skull. These are frontal, parietal, temporal, and occipital lobes. The term cerebrum refers to the areas that overlap from the frontal into the parietal area. All of these lobes are paired (one on each side). There is no clear demarcation of each lobe when looking at the superficial brain surface.

Within the brain are ventricles, areas that act as reservoirs for cerebrospinal fluid. They are numbered and drain different areas of the brain depending on their location (see Figure 6.4).

The bulk of the brain is composed of the cerebral cortex, which forms most of the dorsorostral area. A small protuberance at the rostral cerebrum is the olfactory bulb, which is involved in the sense of smell. The cerebrum has two longitudinal halves called hemispheres. There is a connection between them known as the corpus callosum, which helps transfer information from one side of the brain to the other.

Caudal to the cerebrum is a rounded structure known as the cerebellum. Making a longitudinal incision of this area will reveal a series of channels that resemble the branches of a tree. These structures are collectively referred to as the arbor vitae (trees of life) and are the white matter tracts within this part of the brain. Ventral to the cerebellum is the brain stem, which tapers at its caudal point to become the spinal cord. Many of the cranial nerves arise from the brain stem. Along the ventral surface of the brain stem is the pons. Its name reflects the Latin root word meaning bridge. This area bridges the cerebrum and the cerebellum (Figure 6.2).

The cranial nerves are nerve cell bundles, each of which serves one or more specific functions. Their names are associated with their target (the part of the body they aim toward) or their function. See Box 6.1 for their names and numbers; note that we use Roman numerals to denote the numbers.

Cranial nerve I, the olfactory nerve, runs between the olfactory bulb and the nasal cavity. The optic nerve, cranial nerve II, arises at the retina of each eye and travels toward the brain. It is clearly seen on the ventral surface of the brain (Figure 18.3). The area where some of the nerve fibers from each eye cross to the opposite side of the brain is called the optic chiasm. The largest of the cranial nerves is the trigeminal, and the longest is the vagus. The vagus travels almost the entire length of the body and

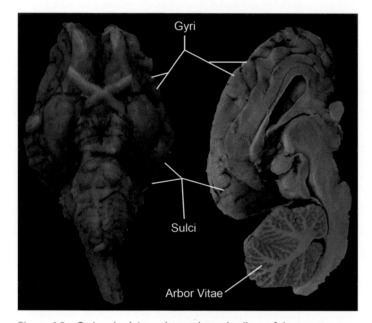

Figure 6.3   Gyri and sulci are the peaks and valleys of the outer surface of the brain. Section of the cerebellum reveals nerve pathways referred to as the arbor vitae (tree of life).

Box 6.1   The cranial nerves

I: olfactory	VII: facial
II: optic	VIII: vestibulocochlear
III: oculomotor	IX: glossopharyngeal
IV: trochlear	X: vagus
V: trigeminal	XI: spinal accessory
VI: abducens	XII: hypoglossal

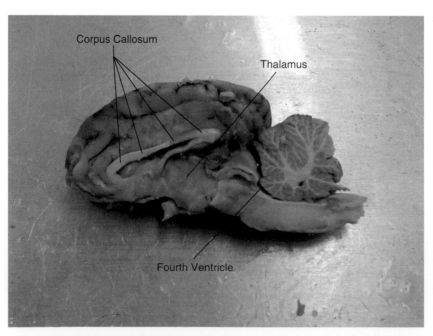

Figure 6.4   Some of the structures of the interior of the brain. The corpus callosum is the connection between the hemispheres. The fourth ventricle is an area that normally is filled with cerebrospinal fluid.

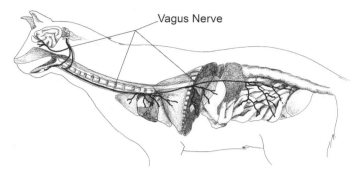

Vagus Nerve

Figure 6.5   The vagus nerve (from the Latin root word for "wanderer") is the longest nerve of the body. It is cranial nerve X and is one of the major carriers of information for the autonomic nervous system.

is the mediator of the autonomic nervous system (see Figure 6.5). We will discuss this at greater length in the physiology section.

The spinal cord

The brain stem narrows as it runs caudally, but it widens again slightly as it approaches the foramen magnum. This swelling is known as the medulla oblongata and is considered to be the cranial origin of the spinal cord. The spinal cord has meninges. They are the same as in the brain with one exception. Superficial to the dura, between the dura mater and the wall of the spinal canal, is a space. It is called the epidural space. The epidural space is an area in which local anesthetic is often injected prior to surgical procedures in the area.

The body of the spinal cord consists of white matter, with a gray matter core. This is the opposite of brain structure, in which the gray matter is on the outside and the white matter lies deep to it. (The structure "turns inside out" so that the gray matter is interior, after the pons). On the transverse section of the spinal cord, the gray matter is shaped like a butterfly. Nerves enter and exit the spinal cord as a trunk called the dorsal or ventral root. There is one on each side, in (not surprisingly) the dorsal or ventral area of the cord. See Figure 18.1 for a schematic drawing of a section of the spinal cord.

The spinal cord does not go all the way through the body to the end of the tail. In the area of the sacrum, the spinal cord fans out into a series of smaller nerves. This area is known as the cauda equina—literally, horse's tail—which it resembles. Peripheral nerves radiate out from this area.

Peripheral nervous system

A plexus is an interlacing series of multiple nerve fiber junctions (not neuronal bodies, which is what distinguishes it from a ganglion). There is a cervical plexus that involves many of the nerves supplying the neck and diaphragm. There is also the brachial plexus, a large area of nerves serving the thoracic limb. It is easily seen in the area of the axilla (where the thoracic limb meets the body) once the surrounding musculature is reflected. Another major plexus is the lumbar plexus.

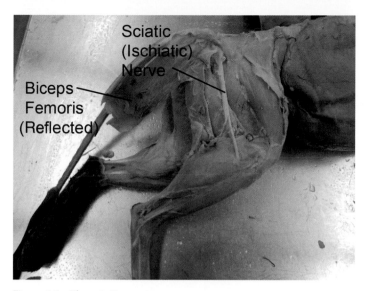

Sciatic (Ischiatic) Nerve

Biceps Femoris (Reflected)

Figure 6.6   The sciatic nerve.

Nerves supplying the head include many of the cranial nerves; one-third of them have some specific function related to the eye. The trigeminal nerve runs in part along the mandible. The auriculopalpebral nerve is a branch of the facial nerve and courses in an area around the rostral pinna and the eyes. It is a convenient place to deliver an analgesic medication when doing eye surgery.

In the thoracic limb, there are a few nerves of major import. The radial nerve runs along the lateral surface all the way to the paw. This nerve is the one that is responsible for the pain response when blood is taken from the thoracic limb (usually, from the cephalic vein). The median nerve runs along the medial surface, dividing into medial and lateral branches at the paw. A tourniquet that is too tight may compress either of these nerves to the point where damage occurs. In this case, given that these nerves affect the entire limb, significant lameness will result. The ulnar nerve also runs along the medial surface of the antebrachium toward the paw.

The pelvic limb has several major nerves. The femoral nerve arises directly from the spinal cord and supplies much of the medial femoral area. The saphenous nerve arises from the cranial femoral nerve and continues to run distally to the tarsus.

The ischiatic or sciatic nerve is very thick and is easily located deep to the muscles biceps femoris and semitendinosus (see Figure 6.6). It innervates much of the pelvic limb. It is very important to avoid impinging on this nerve when giving an intramuscular injection. Some people avoid the problem entirely by using the cranial rather than the caudal thigh when giving an injection. Damage to this nerve can, at worst, cause complete loss of function of the limb.

The pudendal nerve arises from the area of the sacrum and has an impact on the pelvis, genitalia, rectum, and perineum. One of its branches is the caudal rectal nerve. This nerve supplies the external anal sphincter. Any surgery in the area of the rectum needs to be done avoiding this nerve. The consequence of damaging it can be incontinence for feces. A surgery done in this area might be removal of the anal sacs (sebaceous glands on either side of the anus) or repair of a perineal fistula (an opening into the body in the area of the anus, lateral to it).

Clinical case resolution: Intramuscular injection

It is now clear why many people avoid injecting into the area of the semitendinosus. As the sciatic nerve ventures relatively close to it, there is a risk of penetrating the nerve. It innervates most of the limb; therefore, the further away from it, the better.

Review questions

1 What are the two major nerves of the antebrachium?
2 Define the term ganglion.
3 What is the name of cranial nerve XI?
4 What gives white matter its color?
5 What is the proper name of the sciatic nerve?
6 Which layer of the meninges is present in the spinal cord but not in the brain?
7 Where does the spinal cord connect with the brain?
8 Where would you sample cerebrospinal fluid?
9 What nerve would you anesthetize before ophthalmic surgery?
10 What is a bundle of nerve fibers called?

Chapter **7** **Anatomy of the Urinary Tract**

Clinical case: Cat with increased urination and weight loss

A client brings a cat into the clinic which has been urinating outside the litter box, producing a large volume of urine, and drinking more water than he normally does. The cat has lost weight and is inappetent. The client is considering euthanizing the animal. Permission is given to do bloodwork and a urinalysis. The diagnosis becomes apparent with the information from the laboratory assessment of the blood and urine.

Introduction

The above scenario is encountered often in clinical practice. Dogs and cats have a urinary system similar to that of humans in structure and function, but there are important differences. The cat in particular has variations in structure that set the scene for some of the most common illnesses encountered, particularly in older animals.

The kidneys

Physiologically complex, the urinary system can be said to begin with the kidneys (see Figure 7.1). In dogs and cats, there are two, one on each side of the animal. They reside in the dorsal abdomen, approximately deep to the cranial lumbar vertebrae. The right kidney lies cranially in the abdomen relative to the left kidney. This spatial difference reflects the position of the heart toward the left of the midline, only leaving room for the left kidney more caudally. The cranial and caudal borders of the kidneys are called the cranial and caudal poles. The cranial pole of the right kidney is nestled against a hepatic fossa (a shallow depression, so named because it resembles the fossa of a bone). It is in a more fixed position as a result of this, compared with the left kidney.

In most species of mammals, the kidneys rest in the retroperitoneal cavity, which is to say dorsal to the peritoneal membrane that surround the abdominal cavity and most of its internal organs. They generally can be palpated with firm exploration of the cranial abdomen in smaller animals. The outer surface is often surrounded by a layer or partial layer of fat.

Anatomy and Physiology for Veterinary Technicians and Nurses: A Clinical Approach, First Edition. Robin Sturtz and Lori Asprea.
© 2012 John Wiley & Sons, Inc. Published 2012 by John Wiley & Sons, Inc.

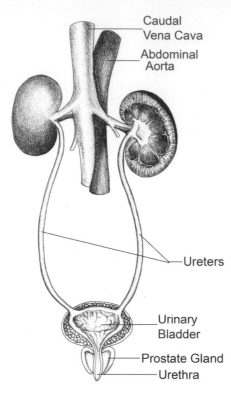

Figure 7.1   The general structure of the urinary system, which starts at the kidney and ends at the distal urethra. While this drawing is of a male (the prostate gland is only found in males), the female architecture is similar. Notice that the interior of the urinary bladder is wrinkled. This gives it extra surface area so that it can expand and contract.

The superficial surface of the kidney is covered by a capsule composed of fibrous material. In life, it has a dark red/brown color. Its shape is that of an oval with an indentation on the medial surface. This forms the derivation of the name of the kidney bean. This indentation is known as the hilus and is the point of entry and exit for the renal artery and vein, as well as the ureter. Note that not all mammals have kidneys in this shape. For example, the dolphin kidney resembles a cluster of grapes. The kidney of the horse has a Valentine heart shape, and that of the bovine is lobed.

The best manner in which to view the kidney is to leave the abdominal viscera attached to the body and to shift them toward the midline to reveal the kidney. The artery and vein are easily visualized. The ureter will have an off-white appearance and resembles a flat strand of spaghetti. Sever the left kidney from these vessels at the hilus, leaving the right kidney in position. The kidney can be most easily transected and its deeper structure viewed in this manner. Once the kidney is extracted from the body, remove the renal capsule and make a longitudinal incision to reveal the interior of each half of the kidney.

Note that craniomedially to the kidney within the abdominal cavity is a small, flat, pink/gray organ with a somewhat rounded shape. This is the adrenal gland. Do not remove it at this time.

On the surface of the kidney, a large number of vessels are noted. In its role as the filter of all the blood in the body, its

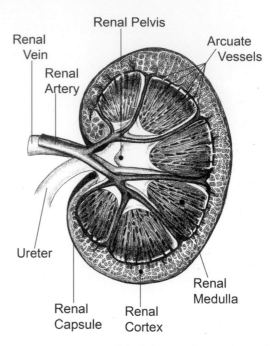

Figure 7.2   Interior structure of the kidney. In dogs and cats, the kidney is surrounded by a capsule. The body wall is to the right in this image, and the head is toward the top of the page.

vascularization is complex. The interior layer of the kidney just deep to the capsule is referred to as the renal cortex (see Figure 7.2). It is a relatively narrow, brick-red area that has a granular appearance. (It may appear beige in a preserved specimen.) Its deeper border has a scalloped appearance. This border is referred to as the corticomedullary boundary. Deep to this boundary is the renal medulla. It is a darker red and has a striated appearance. It has a much larger surface area than the cortex. Toward the hilus, it will take on a gray appearance.

The functional unit of the kidney is a microscopic structure called the nephron. It will be discussed at greater length in the physiology section of this text. Note for the moment that the nephron travels between the cortex and the medulla and that, while there are many nephrons in all mammals, the exact number is species specific. For example, the cat has fewer nephrons than other mammals.

As the microscopic parts of the functional structures of the kidney course through the medulla, they fan out into a dilated area that is concave and whitish gray in color. This area is known as the renal pelvis. (Note again the importance of proper terminology. The *pelvis* is a bony structure; the *renal pelvis* is soft tissue.) Filtrate collects in the renal pelvis and is funneled into the ureter. As the liquid filtered by the kidney exits via the ureter, it is referred to as urine.

Leaving the kidney

The ureter exits the kidney at the hilus and continues along the dorsal retroperitoneal cavity toward the urinary bladder. It curves medially, entering a connective tissue sheet called the genital fold in the male and the broad ligament in the female. The ureter enters the urinary bladder on its dorsal surface, near the neck of the urinary bladder. On rare occasions, the ureter enters in an abnormal place; this condition is known as ectopic ureter. Bear in mind that there will be a ureter entering the urinary bladder from each side. The ureter enters at an angle, which helps discourage the reflux of urine out of the urinary bladder when the bladder contracts.

In the female, the ureter runs alongside the oviduct (the connection between the ovary and the uterus). This is particularly important to keep in mind during ovariohysterectomy ("spay"). Severing the ureter instead of the oviduct will result in life-threatening injury. The surgeon will be careful to trace the structure carefully toward the ovary before incising it.

The ureter contains a layer of smooth muscle. The contraction of this muscle can help expel urine. It can also go into painful spasm in certain conditions, such as when a calculus (stone) is present within it.

The urinary bladder

The urinary bladder is an oval, hollow organ that will have a gray appearance on dissection. Be cautious on incising the bladder; it may contain urine even after the death of the animal. Note the use of the phrase "urinary bladder." As there is another structure called a gallbladder in dogs and cats, the use of the single word "bladder" is imprecise.

In life, the urinary bladder is distensible and is found in the caudal abdomen. The cranial-most part of the urinary bladder is quite mobile; this allows it to fill with urine to a greater or lesser extent depending on the amount of liquid material involved. The fact that the position and size of the urinary bladder can vary means that it is very important to locate it exactly before performing cystocentesis during a physical exam. Blindly placing a needle into the abdomen in an attempt to extract urine may cause the examiner to perforate the intestine or a blood vessel. The apex of the urinary bladder may have a short blind tunnel (a diverticulum). This is the remnant of a fetal vessel (the urachus). It is possible to have material, such as calculi (plural of calculus), trapped in this area. The entire urinary bladder is suspended from the dorsal abdomen by the round ligament, a fibrous tissue that is in part the remnant of the umbilical artery.

The caudal section becomes quite narrow, and it is also referred to as the neck of the urinary bladder.

In the female, the urinary bladder is connected with the broad ligament, which also attaches to the uterus. In the male, the urinary bladder is within the genital fold of the membrane, which also contains the ductus deferens (a conduit for sperm, which will be discussed in the chapter on reproductive anatomy).

The urinary bladder has a strong muscular coat. The detrusor muscle has a particularly important role in urinary physiology. The urethralis muscle also has such a role.

The muscles that form the gateway between the urinary bladder and the urethra, a sphincter, have both skeletal and smooth muscle components. As such, there is both voluntary and involuntary control over the opening of the sphincter and, thus, of urination. Injury to the muscles or the nerves controlling them contributes to urinary incontinence, which is when the animal urinates when or where it ordinarily should not.

The urinary bladder has a number of layers on a microscopic level. One of the layers of the interior epithelium is a type of cell called a transitional cell. Seen more in dogs than in cats, transitional cell carcinoma is the most common cancer of the urinary bladder.

Careful examination of the interior surface of the urinary bladder in the area of the neck may reveal three small openings. Two of these are the entrances of the right and left ureters. The other is the exit for urine as it enters the urethra. This area is the trigone and is the site of most transitional cell carcinomas.

As urine exits the urinary bladder, it enters the urethra, which leads to the outside of the body. This area will be difficult to uncover during dissection without fracturing or disassembling the pelvis; if observation *in situ* is desired, it is best to wait until all other dissection has been completed in order to view it.

In the female, the urethra runs along the ventral pelvis and is ventral to the reproductive tract. It passes into the vagina at the vestibular junction and becomes one passage toward the outside. As the urethra rises dorsally to make this entrance, and because there can be a small turn in the vagina in that area, the placement of a urinary catheter in a female dog or cat is usually difficult. Substantial practice is required to do this effectively. The urethra is surrounded by the urethralis muscle and is innervated by the pudendal nerve. Its submucosal tissue has erectile tissue, which also contributes to continence. Otherwise, its structure is similar to that of the urinary bladder.

In the male, the urethra exits the urinary bladder and enters the penis (see Figure 7.3). The pelvic part of the urethra is the

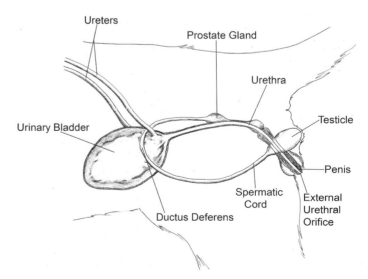

Figure 7.3   Note that in male cats, the urethra actually curves as it passes the prostate to head toward the penis. Mucus, particles, or other solid matter can become trapped there, causing a potentially life-threatening obstruction.

section of it within the body. As the urethra exits the body, it is referred to as the external urethra. It is surrounded by spongy tissue as it travels the length of the penis. In the pelvic urethra, near the urinary bladder, it is joined by the reproductive ducts. This area is referred to as the colliculus. This junction explains why the penis is able to discharge both urine and semen. The dorsal surface of the pelvic urethra is just deep to the rectum. For this reason, palpation of the rectum can cause muscular contraction of the urethra.

The course of the urethra in the male cat is a unique one. The cat is the only mammal whose penis faces caudally. Therefore, as the urethra extends away from the urinary bladder, it travels in a circuitous route, running caudally, then cranially, then caudally again. This curve can cause material to become trapped if there is particulate matter (such as calculi) or mucus plugs. This results in obstruction of the urethra and causes urine to back up toward the urinary bladder.

The avian system is quite different. From the kidney, waste material is transported to a central area in the caudal abdomen known as the cloaca. "Urine" is not actually liquid in the avian but is composed of urea-loaded crystals. The cloaca also accepts fecal material from the digestive tract. As a result, renal and digestive excreta exit from the same location in the animal. In fact, the egg also exits by way of the cloaca.

The blocked cat

The condition of urethral obstruction is commonly referred to as "blocked cat." This can become fatal in as little as 1 day. Clients should always be cautioned that if their male cat does not urinate at least once in 24 hours, they should bring the patient in for examination. Usually, the abdomen will feel rigid, and radiography will reveal a large urinary bladder that may extend cranially to a position past the mid-abdomen. Rapid placement of a urinary catheter and fluid therapy are crucial.

Clinical case resolution: Cat with increased urination and weight loss

The cat has fewer nephrons than any other mammal. As a result, normal wear and tear over time causes a problem in felines more often than in canines. Kidney disease is one of the most common health problems in older cats. Dysfunction of the kidney causes liquid to be excreted rather than reserved, even though the fluid might be needed. The animal becomes dehydrated. The central nervous system tries to redress the balance by directing the animal to drink more. The kidney cannot reserve the liquid, however, so urine volume increases. The animal can become even more dehydrated, even though fluid intake has increased. The large volume of urine puts pressure on the urinary bladder, and the animal feels the urge to void so strongly that he or she cannot wait until the litter box is near. The condition is uncomfortable, and the patient often becomes anorexic.

The above explains all of the signs noted at the outset of this chapter. The bloodwork reveals kidney dysfunction, and the urinalysis reveals the urine to have a high protein content, which is common in kidney disease. Treatment strategies have been studied extensively and have variable outcomes.

Review questions

1 Which is deeper, the renal cortex or the renal medulla?
2 What is the name of the indentation in the kidney from which the ureter comes?
3 True or false: In the dog and cat, the kidney is covered by a fibrous capsule.
4 On what surface of the urinary bladder does the ureter enter?
5 What is unusual about the structure of the feline male urethra?

Chapter **8** **Cardiovascular Anatomy**

Clinical case: Norwegian forest cat

A Norwegian Forest cat is brought into the clinic for an examination. A clear murmur is noted on ausculting the heart sounds. Radiography suggests that the heart size is larger than normal. How does this relate to the heart murmur? Why does the breed of cat matter?

Introduction

The circulatory system includes a number of structures and vessels. The heart, veins, arteries, and lymphatic vessels play a role in the passage of fluids throughout the body. They are aided by lymph nodes and (indirectly) by the spleen and the thymus. All of these organs and conduits have the same goal: to bring needed materials (oxygen, nutrients, inflammatory cells, platelets) throughout the animal and to remove waste products (carbon dioxide, cell debris, interstitial fluid). These processes will be discussed at greater length in Chapter 20.

The heart

The heart is a large organ within the thoracic cavity, situated near the midline, between the left and right lung lobes. It is covered by a connective tissue sac called the pericardium. The pericardium is composed of three layers. The superficial layer is called the fibrous pericardium. Deep to this is a two-layered membrane that forms the serous pericardium. The parietal layer is superficial to the visceral layer, which actually adheres to and combines with the outer surface of the heart (the epicardium). Between the layers of the serous pericardium is a small amount (less than 1 mL) of viscous fluid. In certain cardiac diseases or cardiac malfunction, excess fluid forms within the pericardium, and the increased pressure can then itself interfere with heart function. This condition is called pericardial effusion and makes the heart sound muffled on auscultation. The sac can be surgically fenestrated or even removed without significant consequences in order to decrease the pressure against the heart.

Deep to the epicardium is the myocardium, the actual heart muscle. It has a unique microscopic structure, partly like smooth muscle and partly like skeletal muscle. The myocardial layer is thicker in some areas than in others. In particular, the area

Anatomy and Physiology for Veterinary Technicians and Nurses: A Clinical Approach, First Edition. Robin Sturtz and Lori Asprea.
© 2012 John Wiley & Sons, Inc. Published 2012 by John Wiley & Sons, Inc.

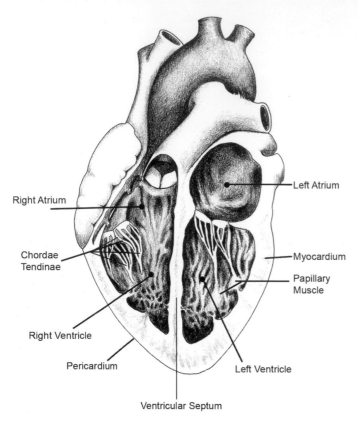

Figure 8.1   Chambers of the heart. Notice that the wall of the left ventricle is slightly thicker than that of the right ventricle. This relates to the greater force required of the left ventricle on contraction of the heart.

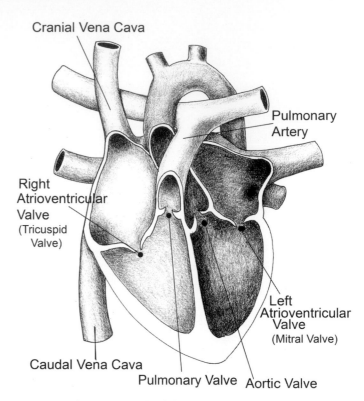

Figure 8.2   The great vessels of the heart and the major valves. The aortic and pulmonary valves are referred to as semilunar valves because of their reported resemblance to the shape of the crescent moon.

around the left ventricle is much thicker. The endocardium is the lining of the interior chambers of the heart. It is contiguous with, and in fact becomes, the lining of some of the great vessels, such as the aorta.

In mammals, the heart has four chambers: a right atrium, left atrium, right ventricle, and left ventricle (see Figure 8.1). Looking at the animal in dorsal recumbency, the atria are cranial to the ventricles. The wider part of the heart is cranial to the narrower part. The wider portion is the base of the heart, and the thinner end is the apex. The great vessels are the aorta, pulmonary arteries, pulmonary veins, cranial vena cava, and caudal vena cava. As can be seen in Figure 8.2, the basic circulation into and through the heart involves blood leaving the left ventricle via the aorta, passing through other arteries throughout the body, and then returning to the heart by way of a number of veins that feed into the cranial and caudal vena cava (plural form: cavae). The vena cavae enter the right atrium of the heart. Blood flows into the right ventricle and is carried toward the lungs by the pulmonary trunk (pulmonary artery). Blood is thus transported to the lungs and oxygenated. It then is transported to the left atrium by way of the pulmonary veins. Blood travels from there to the left ventricle, and the cycle continues.

The heart itself has a circulatory system as well (see Figure 8.3). Coronary arteries and veins supply the heart muscle and

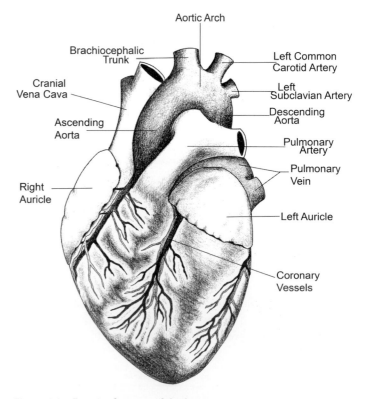

Figure 8.3   Exterior features of the heart.

support structures and are visible on the heart once the pericardium has been removed.

The heart is present in most vertebrate circulatory systems, but there is, as usual, a great deal of species differentiation. The heart of the dogfish has only two main chambers and two great vessels (one artery, one vein). Snakes and other reptiles have a three-chambered heart.

The exterior of the heart

Upon severing the ribs from the sternebrae on one side of the thorax, the heart will be revealed, nestled between the right and left lung lobes. The thickest vessel at the base of the heart, which travels a short distance cranially before turning and continuing caudally, is the aorta. It is the artery that gives rise to almost all of the others that course through the body. Note that arteries are vessels that travel away from the heart, and veins are those that travel to the heart. On the exterior surface of the heart, two "leaves" can be seen near the base, in the area of the pulmonary trunk. These structures are known as auricles, from the root word for "ear." You may also see a small cord of fibrous tissue connecting the pulmonary trunk and the aorta. This is called the ligamentum arteriosum. It is the remnant of a fetal vessel, the ductus arteriosus, that brings blood directly from the heart to the arteries without visiting the lungs. If the duct does not close properly once the puppy or kitten is born, blood cannot be oxygenated properly. This birth defect is found most often in certain dog breeds and is known as patent ductus arteriosus (PDA).

The interior of the heart

Dissect the heart along the long axis, along its midline. Four chambers are revealed. The ventricles are longer than the atria and sit caudal to the atria. Separating the atrium from the ventricle on each side is a fibrous structure known as an atrioventricular valve. On the right side of the heart, the atrioventricular valve is known as the tricuspid valve. It actually only has two cusps (leaves) in the dog. The left atrioventricular valve is known as the mitral valve, as it supposedly resembles a bishop's hat (miter). Supporting these valves are two structures: papillary muscles and chorda tendinae. The papillary muscles are anchored in the endocardium. The chordae tendinae are fibrous strands that have tremendous tensile strength. In ruminants and in older horses, there is actually a bony attachment to the valves called the os cordis.

The entrances to the aorta and the pulmonary trunk are also covered by valves. The leaflets are considered to resemble a half-moon and are referred to as semilunar valves. The aortic valve has three cusps, while the pulmonary has only two.

Dividing the left and right sides of the heart is a thickened wall called the coronary septum. The cranial part of the wall (between the atria, referred to as the interatrial septum) is relatively thin. In the fetus, there is an opening in the septum between the atria called the foramen ovale. It closes abruptly when the infant is born. If it does not close properly, the condition is called atrial septal defect. It, too, is somewhat common in certain dog breeds. A more serious condition, ventricular septal defect, is much less common.

The heart moves blood toward the lungs from the right ventricle. This is the beginning of what is called the pulmonary circuit. The left ventricle launches blood toward the rest of the body, referred to as the systemic circuit. As can be imagined, a great deal more force is needed to launch blood throughout the body. Therefore, it is not surprising that the left ventricular wall is thicker than the right wall, and the aortic valve is thicker than the pulmonary valve.

When looking at a dog or a cat during a physical exam, the heart can be visualized as extending from the second or third intercostal space to the fifth or sixth intercostal space, about two-thirds of the way up from the sternum. In auscultating the heart on the left side of the body, sounds associated with the mitral valve can be best heard at the fifth intercostal space, at the level of the olecranon. The pulmonary valve can be heard at the third intercostal space, at the same level. The aortic valve is best heard at the fourth intercostal space, near the shoulder. In order to remember this architecture, some use the device PAM left, T right (pulmonary, aortic, mitral on the left side, then tricuspid on the right side of the animal).

Peripheral circulation

The rest of the circulatory system consists of vessels that carry blood or other fluid throughout the body. Most often, the smallest of the arteries and veins are connected via very narrow vessels called capillaries. There are occasions where arteries connect to each other directly. These are called anastomoses and allow multiple arteries to serve a given area.

Arteries tend to course in protected areas, deep within the trunk or on the medial surface of the limbs. Their route is often circuitous. Small arteries are referred to as arterioles. The largest of the arteries is the aorta, which arises directly from the left ventricle of the heart. Most of the larger branches of the aorta divide off at an angle to it in order to decrease some of the force of the blood flow; the strong pulse is a direct reflection of the fact that the aorta exits the heart itself, rather than branching from another vessel.

While veins have thinner walls, they generally have a greater diameter and/or capacity to carry blood (with the exception of the aorta). The smallest veins are called venules. Unlike arteries, most veins of the trunk and limbs have valves within their lumen, composed of two or three semilunar cusps. These help keep blood flow unidirectional.

The other major type of vessel is the lymphatic vessel. These mostly arise from a group of capillaries called a venous plexus (in order to distinguish it from a nerve plexus). The lymphatic vessels have the capacity to pick up larger molecules (such as proteins) and other particulate matter that has ended up in the interstitial fluid (the interstitial area is the material between the cells). The lymphatic vessels have closely spaced valves, and sometimes will have a beaded appearance. Unlike arteries and veins, lymphatic vessels start off very small and become larger as they travel. Eventually, they form major vessels, or trunks, which eventually empty into veins.

Many lymphatic vessels pass through a lymph node as they travel. These are firm, smooth structures covered by a capsule (thin "overcoat"). In the carnivore, there are relatively few lymph nodes, but they are large and tend to be found in clusters. In contrast, equines have small lymph nodes but spread all over the body. In dogs and cats, a number of lymphatic vessels will enter the node at once, but material exits the node in one vessel. The function of these nodes will be discussed later. For now, note that in an animal who has active inflammatory disease, these nodes may appear quite large; this is referred to as a reactive node. The nodes can also be enlarged in other disease states, such as the cancer known as lymphoma.

A tonsil is a special type of lymph node. Tonsils do not have a capsule and are generally not associated with lymphatic vessels. They occur in the pharynx, genitals, and intestines, and are available to filter contaminated material away from the area.

Certain lymph nodes can be palpated during a physical exam. In dogs, we can check the submandibular, prescapular, axillary, inguinal, and popliteal lymph nodes. The submandibulars are ventral to the caudal mandible. The prescapulars are in the cranial thorax, close to where the trunk meets the leg. The popliteal lymph nodes are found just caudal to the stifle. These nodes are so close to the surface that they are readily palpable. In cats, the popliteal lymph node is not generally palpable unless it is responding to disease. In bovines, you may be able to palpate the prescapular nodes.

The layers of arteries are called tunics (from the Latin word for covering). The outermost layer is a fibrous coat of connective tissue, which protects against excessive expansion and possible rupture. The middle layer is the thickest and consists of elastic tissues and occasional stretches of smooth muscle. The innermost layer is the endothelium, which consists of elastic connective tissue as well as epithelial cells. The connective tissue in the arteries of domestic animals does not generally become very stiff; in humans, however, this is common with age and is informally called "hardening" of the arteries (atherosclerosis). The open space at the center of a hollow vessel or organ is called a lumen. Thus, the luminal surface is the one that is innermost, lining the "hole" through the center of the vessel (or organ, such as the interior of the intestine, gallbladder, or urinary bladder).

The arteries arising directly from the heart, and some of their major branches, are mostly elastic tissue, with little or no muscle in the middle tunic. Note that the pulmonary trunk, which arises from the right ventricle of the heart and heads toward the lungs, is an artery. The term artery refers not to oxygen content but to whether or not blood is flowing away from the heart or not.

Not all arteries have specific names. Some named arteries have more muscle tissue. Contraction of these muscles can decrease the diameter of the vessel and helps control the pressure of the blood flow. This is called vasoconstriction.

The arteries become capillaries, which are small, narrow vessels that are extensions of the endothelial tissue, with a delicate connective tissue covering. Some fluid passes from the capillaries into the interstitium, and some transfers directly to the veins. Some capillaries, particularly in the intestines and part of the kidney, are fenestrated (have small window-like pores allowing the exit or entrance of larger molecules). Sinusoids, which are wider, and often fenestrated, groups of capillaries, can actually take in very large particles. Sinusoids are found in the liver, the spleen, and the bone marrow.

In contrast to most arteries, the outer tunic of veins is mostly elastic connective tissue, with the middle layer mostly muscle. The endothelium is thin, with no elastic tissue. Folds that descend into the lumen of the vessel form the valves.

Given that the vessels are composed of living tissue, they themselves need a blood supply. Small vessels called the vasa vasorum supply the blood vessels with a blood supply of their own.

The blood vessels have extensive innervation. Among other functions, these nerves help control blood pressure. They will be discussed in Chapter 20.

A group of arterioles can form anastomoses, as noted above. These structures, in turn, can form a network (cluster) called a rete. The best-known rete is the renal glomerulus, a part of the nephron.

Many animals presented for classroom necropsy have been injected with a silicone-based material to make the vessels stand out. By convention, the arteries are colored red and the veins blue. Occasionally, excessive force is used in injecting the dye, leading to large clumps of plastic appearing within the vasculature or to a lack of coloring in the distal vessels. This is a post-mortem phenomenon and does not represent pathology.

The named arteries

As the aorta exits the heart itself, it has a widened appearance, referred to as the aortic bulb. It can be identified nestled between the atria, approximately above the area of the mitral valve. The coronary arteries arise from the aortic bulb, supplying the heart itself with oxygen. As the aorta exits the pericardium, it travels cranially and is called the ascending aorta. The part that starts to bend around is called the aortic arch. Arteries leading from the aortic arch include such major vessels as the brachiocephalic trunk, the left subclavian artery, and the common carotid artery (see Figure 8.4).

The carotid artery splits into left and right carotids, which travel all the way to the brain. There is an external carotid and an internal carotid on each side, which diverge approximately at the level of the larynx. The internal carotid, protected by being deep within the body, goes directly to the brain. The external carotid has a number of branches that supply other areas of the neck and head. These include the facial artery, which runs along the mandible. Other branches include the maxillary artery, supplying the teeth and eye, and the superficial maxillary artery, supplying the masseter muscle and the eyelids.

The carotids, if occluded, will choke off the supply of oxygen, glucose, and other materials the brain needs to stay alive. As is true for all major arteries, they have a pulsing movement that reflects the heart pumping the blood along. In dogs and cats, the carotid artery is one vessel we use to check the pulse. (In the

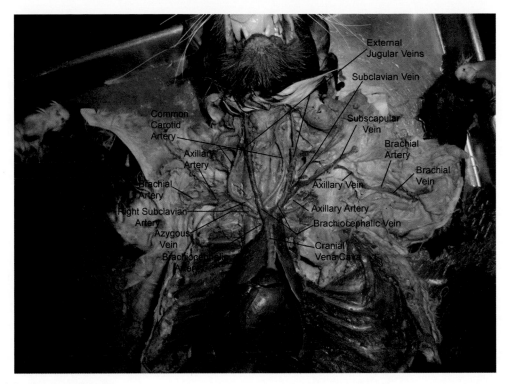

Figure 8.4   Vessels of the thorax and neck.

horse, where this vessel is not accessible, we use the facial artery instead, easily felt ventral and slightly medial to the lateral mandible) We often take blood samples from the jugular vein of a dog or cat, which also runs through the neck. Observe the vessel you are planning to sample blood from carefully; if it is pulsing, plunging a needle into it can cause the animal to lose a great deal of blood.

The subclavian artery diverges into a number of branches. The vertebral artery moves cranially to supply the spinal cord and brain. Another branch is the internal thoracic artery, which courses caudally and becomes the cranial epigastric artery.

The internal thoracic artery may be hard to locate on dissection. The epigastric artery assumes importance in large-scale skin grafts, such as after a burn injury; the artery is often diverted to provide blood to the grafted skin.

The subclavian artery also courses along to the axilla (essentially, the armpit), where it is called the axillary artery. It continues distally along the medial brachium to the cranial elbow, where it becomes the median artery. It gives off a number of branches, including one called the superficial brachial artery. This artery is important in that it runs along the cephalic vein and radial nerve. The cephalic vein is one of the most commonly used vessels for routine phlebotomy in the dog. It is important to avoid the nearby artery during this procedure. Other branches continue toward the paw.

In dissecting into the axilla, a tangle of vessels and nerves will be noted. The nerves are off-white in color and resist breaking even when tugged firmly. This nest is called the brachial plexus. Again, since there are so many important vessels and nerves, it is no surprise that it is in such a protected area.

After giving off the major vessels, the aorta executes a turn and begins to course caudally. Once this happens, it is referred to as the descending aorta. The thoracic section runs next to the azygous vein and the thoracic duct (a major lymphatic vessel) and enters the abdomen through a hole in the diaphragm called the aortic hiatus. The abdominal section of the aorta continues caudally to the area of the caudal lumbar vertebrae, where it branches into two major arteries. There is a pair of external iliac arteries and a pair of internal iliac arteries. The aorta does continue past this point, but here it is a very thin vessel called the median sacral artery, which supplies the tail (see Figure 8.5).

The fork at the distal aorta, where the iliac arteries branch off, is an important landmark. In cats, where a blood clot forms in the heart or in the arterial system, the clot will travel along the aorta and come to rest at this fork. This condition is referred to as a saddle thrombus. The clot is unable to move further because of the abrupt change of direction and narrowing of the vessel. Blood supply to the pelvic limbs and tail are cut off. In addition to being extremely painful, this condition is difficult to treat. A cat coming into the clinic showing signs of extreme pain, and whose rear paws are cold, may be suffering from this condition. This is a medical emergency and demands immediate attention.

Returning to the point where the aorta enters the abdomen, the first visceral branch of the abdominal aorta is the celiac artery. The celiac is easily visible on necropsy. It continues to become the hepatic, splenic, and left gastric arteries. The latter supplies the duodenum, the liver and spleen, and the stomach. The hepatic artery branches to the gallbladder, stomach, duodenum, and pancreas.

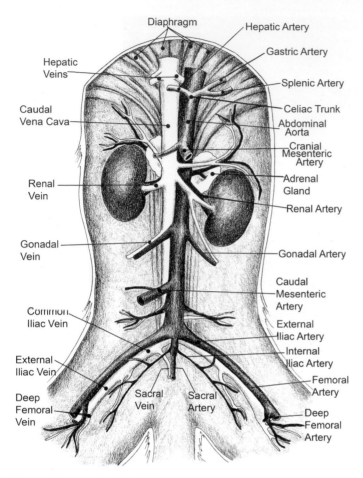

Figure 8.5   Vessels of the abdomen.

The next major artery going caudally is the cranial mesenteric artery. It branches in such a way as to eventually supply the jejunum, ileum, and colon. In this manner, it contributes to the collateral circulation of the intestines. Viewing the mesentery will reveal a network of numerous small arteries. Each section of the small intestine has several arteries supplying oxygen and nutrients. Interruption of any of these arteries thus does not completely deprive any one section of a blood supply. The term "collateral circulation" means that there are many vessels contributing to one area.

Caudal to the cranial mesenteric is the renal artery. This travels directly from the aorta to the kidney. The direct supply from the major artery underscores the importance of the kidney as a filter for the entire bloodstream.

Continuing caudally to a point near the termination of the abdominal aorta is the caudal mesenteric artery, which supplies the colon and the rectum.

As mentioned above, the two caudal-most major branches of the aorta are the external iliac and internal iliac arteries (each one on each side). The external iliac artery is the primary supplier of blood to the hind limb. The deep femoral artery branches off while still within the abdomen. Checking for a pulse is often done using this vessel. In fact, timing the pulse of the femoral artery in contrast to the heartbeat can reveal something

called pulse deficit, an important indicator of circulatory system pathology. Pulse deficit is when the heartbeat and femoral arterial pulse are not synchronized.

The external pudendal artery supplies the groin and prepuce (the tissue surrounding the penis). The femoral artery courses along the medial part of the proximal pelvic limb, then crosses to the caudal part of the limb. It passes caudal to the stifle, where it is called the popliteal artery. This artery, in turn, divides into the cranial and caudal tibial arteries. The cranial tibial artery will be easily found on dissection, but the caudal tibial artery may be more difficult to uncover. The popliteal lymph node will be easily visualized in the fat caudal to the stifle, appearing as a dark, smooth, firm, approximately pea-sized structure.

At the medial midfemoral artery, the saphenous artery branches and continues distally by way of various branches all the way to the paw. The vein, which runs alongside it, called the saphenous vein, is the point where we generally obtain blood samples in cats.

The internal iliac artery brings blood to the pelvic viscera and walls of the caudal abdomen. By way of its branches, it helps supply the urinary bladder (umbilical artery), caudal muscles of the proximal pelvic limb, and gluteal muscles (caudal gluteal artery). The internal pudendal artery branches from the internal iliac artery. Its first branch is the prostatic artery in the male, the vaginal artery in the female. They supply the rectum, urinary bladder and urethra, and the reproductive areas. One branch of the vaginal artery is the ovarian artery.

The veins

The major veins entering the heart are the cranial and caudal vena cavae. The cranial vena cava drains the head and cranial body, and the caudal vena cava the rest of the body. They enter the right atrium of the heart. Blood is carried away from the right ventricle via the pulmonary artery to the lungs. Returning from the lungs with their load of oxygen are the pulmonary veins. The number of these veins varies among species. In dogs, there are two of them; large animals generally have three. The pulmonary veins have no valves. They enter the left atrium. Eventually, the blood enters the left ventricle before being pumped out of the heart.

It is notable that most arteries have a vein paired with them and have essentially the same name. For example, there is a brachiocephalic vein and a brachiocephalic artery. They usually travel next to each other. There are, however, some exceptions.

The aorta does not have a paired vein. Analogous to the aorta is the vena cava; there is no "aortic vein." The same is true for the celiac artery in that there is no celiac vein.

By the time blood starts to return to the heart, it no longer is receiving the strong "push" from the pumping of the heart. Therefore, veins do not pulse as blood moves through them. This plays a role in phlebotomy; if it is pulsing, it is not a vein. We usually sample venous blood for laboratory testing purposes.

Blood returning from the head is carried in the jugular veins (on each side). The jugular vein is often used to obtain a blood sample in dogs and cats. It is the blood vessel we use in almost all cases to obtain blood in equines and bovines as it is readily accessed and big enough to obtain a good sample easily.

The subclavian vein brings blood from the thoracic limbs toward the trunk. One of the distal vessels that feed into the subclavian vein is the cephalic vein. As we mentioned, this is the vein that we use most often to obtain blood from dogs. Both the jugulars and the brachiocephalic veins feed directly into the cranial vena cava.

Coming from the caudal part of the animal, the internal and external iliac veins drain the hind limb and wall of the pelvic area. The external iliac vein is supplied by a vein coming from the crus and femoral part of the limb. This vein is called the median saphenous vein (there is also a lateral saphenous vein). The saphenous vein can be used in dogs to obtain a blood sample but is used most frequently in cats. The iliac veins all feed into the caudal vena cava.

The portal vein eventually receives input from the spleen, digestive organs, rectum, and even the caudal esophagus. This vein plays a major role in the filtering roles of the liver and digestive tract. The renal vein as well as the portal vein eventually feed into the caudal vena cava. As the caudal vena cava tunnels through the liver, it is fed by the hepatic veins.

The azygous vein travels a long course and runs alongside the aorta as it travels into the thorax. It continues cranially and enters the cranial vena cava or the coronary sinus of the right atrium (a shallow bowl where the vena cavae enter the right atrium).

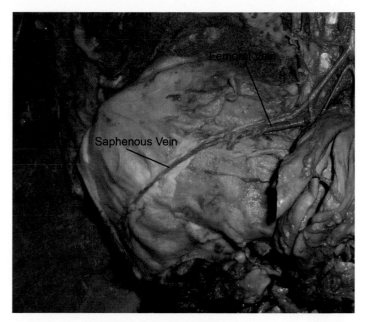

Figure 8.6 The saphenous vein, coursing along the medial thigh. This vessel is commonly used to take a blood sample from a cat.

Box 8.1 **Phlebotomy**

See Figures 8.6 and 8.7.

In order of preference, vessels from which we take blood (the process of drawing blood from a vessel is called phlebotomy) are

Dog: cephalic, saphenous, jugular veins. (We use arterial blood to get blood gas levels, e.g., oxygen.)
Cat: saphenous, cephalic, jugular veins
Equine: jugular

The lymphatic system

Lymph is a fluid that is collected from tissues. It includes white blood cells, occasionally some "used" red blood cells, and interstitial fluid. The thoracic duct is a long vessel that arises in the area of the thoracolumbar junction. It receives lymph from the abdomen as well as the left side of the thorax as it travels cranially. Eventually, it drains into either the left jugular vein or the cranial vena cava. Most lymphatic vessels eventually empty into veins.

Many of the lymphatic vessels pass through lymph nodes, which contribute to the workings of the immune system. Most lymph nodes have a capsular covering. Again, an exception is the tonsils, which are moist, unencapsulated nodules found in the oral, pharyngeal, and intestinal areas.

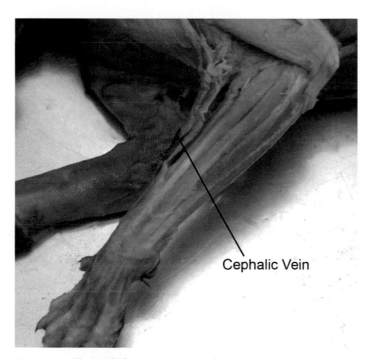

Figure 8.7 The cephalic vein is commonly used to draw blood and to place a venous catheter.

Some of the more important lymph nodes in the cranial body include the parotids (one on each side of the head), the submandibulars (which, among other things, help drain the salivary glands), and the prescapular lymph nodes, which are cranial to the shoulders. There is also a series of lymph nodes in the area of the axilla. There is also a parotid salivary gland, in the area of

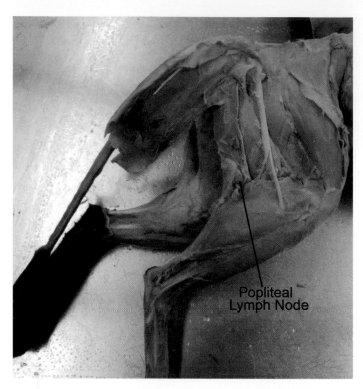

Figure 8.8 The popliteal lymph node is just caudal to the stifle, surrounded by a layer of fat. The biceps femoris is reflected here for better viewing. The animal's head is to the right.

the parotid lymph nodes, so the nomenclature needs particular precision.

Within the thorax, there are several important lymph nodes. There is a dorsal node, a ventral node, and a mediastinal node. The ventral node is just dorsal to the third sternebra. On radiography, it is not usually visible. If a cloudy area is seen at that spot, it may be an enlarged ventral thoracic lymph node; this condition is seen in lymphoma, as well as in severe inflammatory disease. The mediastinal lymph node sits just cranially to the heart, in between the lungs.

The abdomen and the hind limbs contain a number of lymph nodes as well. The popliteal lymph node is the most easily palpated of these (see Figure 8.8). In the caudodorsal abdomen is an area called the ileosacral center, which is a large collection of lymph nodes that serve the abdomen and pelvic cavity.

There are several organs that function as part of the lymphatic circulation or have significant amounts of lymphatic tissue. For example, the spleen contains some tissue called "white pulp." This part receives lymphatic vessels and helps distribute white blood cells throughout the body. The difference in this tissue from the rest of the spleen is microscopic and will not be observed on dissection. The spleen is roughly the shape of an upside-down J when the animal is in dorsal recumbency (lying on his back).

On the animal's left is the head of the spleen. The body of the spleen travels across the body in the area of the stomach. The

tail of the spleen, which is the longest part, is on the animal's right side and is free-floating. The spleen is also mentioned in this chapter because one of its few jobs is to sequester red blood cells and platelets for future use. It is entirely possible for a mammal to exist without one. The spleen can be removed surgically without serious consequence to the animal. This may be done when the animal has suffered severe trauma to the abdomen or when a malignant tumor is present.

There is a great deal of lymphatic drainage from the gastrointestinal (GI) tract. There are areas in the small intestine that are flat and do not have the typical nodular shape. However, these areas, called Peyer's patches, perform the same function as a lymph node.

One other organ of note in this regard is the thymus. The thymus is a structure in the ventral thorax, housed craniolaterally to the heart. It disappears with age; in dogs, it is usually completely atrophied by 2 years of age. On thoracic radiography of a young animal, it has a characteristic sailboat appearance and can be mistaken for a partially collapsed lung lobe.

Clinical case resolution: Norwegian forest cat

We now can understand the problem of the cat mentioned at the beginning of this chapter. The enlargement of the heart will cause it to beat inefficiently. As a result, blood will not flow through in a straight line but will have areas of turbulence. A heart murmur is simply the auditory evidence of turbulent blood flow. The breed of the cat is relevant, in that Norwegian Forest cats have a very high incidence of cardiomyopathy.

Review questions

1 What is the name of the layers of connective tissue that cover the heart?
2 Which chamber of the heart does the aorta come out from?
3 The coronary arteries that feed the heart come from what part of the circulatory system?
4 The vessel exiting toward the lungs from the right ventricle of the heart is the _____.
5 What is the proximal-most branch artery of the abdominal aorta?
6 True or false: The aorta extends all the way down through the tail.
7 The smallest vessels of the arteries, just before they enter the capillaries, are called _____.
8 The major vein that enters the right atrium from the area of the head and neck is the _____.
9 What does the spleen have to do with the circulatory system?
10 What lymph node of the pelvic limb is readily palpable in the dog?

Chapter 9 Anatomy of the Digestive System

Clinical case: Dog with diarrhea and pain

A dog is brought into the clinic with watery diarrhea and severe abdominal pain, particularly in the right cranial quadrant. The location of the pain helps localize the source of the problem. What's the most likely disorder?

Introduction

The anatomy of the digestive tract is amazingly variable among species. The importance of the metabolic processing of food-stuffs dictates examination of the significant differences among them. Dogs and cats will be discussed first. The digestive tract in mammals also includes the liver and pancreas, organs that have digestive and nondigestive functions.

Canines and felines

The alimentary tract is a tube within the body, stretching from the mouth to the anus. There are certain structures that connect to the tract by ducts, such as the salivary glands, the gallbladder, and the pancreas.

In order, from cranial to caudal, the parts include the lips, the teeth and oral cavity, the pharynx, the esophagus, the stomach, the small intestine, the large intestine, the rectum, and the anus. Ancillary structures will be discussed along with each major organ.

The oral cavity

The mouth includes the lips, teeth, tongue, and salivary glands. Note that some of these structures have functions beyond ingestion. These include aggression and defense, conduction of gases to the airway, and amplification of sound.

The outer vestibule of the mouth includes the lips and cheeks, as well as the oral cavity up to the palatoglossal arch, which is the soft tissue border of the caudal oral cavity, approximately at the level of the ramus of the mandible. Depending on the species, the lips can be thick and mobile, or thin and less mobile. They consist of skin, mucosa, nerve endings (supplied mostly by the seventh cranial nerve), and salivary glands. The border between the epidermal and mucosal tissues is referred to as a

Anatomy and Physiology for Veterinary Technicians and Nurses: A Clinical Approach, First Edition. Robin Sturtz and Lori Asprea.
© 2012 John Wiley & Sons, Inc. Published 2012 by John Wiley & Sons, Inc.

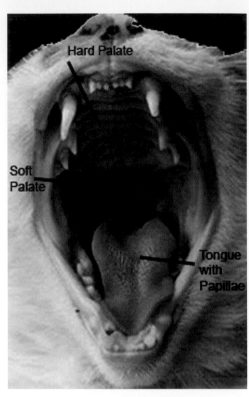

Figure 9.1   The hard palate overlies the palatine bone. Its rugae (ridges) are clearly visible. The soft palate helps guide food down the digestive tract as the food is chewed and swallowed. The papillae are an important part of the sense of taste.

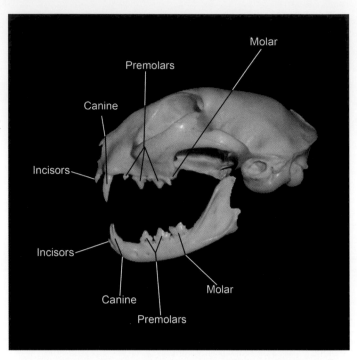

Figure 9.2   Position of the teeth; the upper teeth are rooted in the incisive and maxillary bones, and the lower ones in the mandible. There are no teeth on the ramus of the mandible.

mucocutaneous border. Some of these borders are associated with certain diseases (e.g., lupus erythematosus).

Movement of the ingesta within the oral cavity is assisted by the buccinator muscles within the cheeks. Recall that the temporal and masseter muscles also control this function. The dorsal oral cavity consists of the hard and soft palates. The hard palate covers the ventral palatine bone, while the soft palate does not have a bony backing (see Figure 9.1). The hard palate has ridges, called rugae, which are caudally facing and help direct food further into the digestive tract. The roof of the oral cavity also contains a duct that connects to the nasal cavity. As air passes through this duct, it is conveyed along the nasal cavity to the olfactory mucosa of the vomeronasal organ. This enhances the strength of food odors, which play a large role in the stimulation of appetite. A cat will often, upon encountering an interesting smell, hold his/her mouth open for several seconds to stimulate this organ; this adds to the intensity of the olfactory experience.

The tongue is a mostly muscular feature. The root of the tongue is anchored to the caudal area of the oral cavity and is connected in part to the mandible. The apex of the tongue is the freely mobile, rostral part. Its dorsal surface is covered by thin hairs, composed of connective tissue. It is also the home of small "mounds" of tissue called papillae, which are involved in the sense of taste. Of clinical note: It is important to deflect the root of the tongue ventrally in order to visualize the vocal folds when placing an endotracheal tube.

The salivary glands can either enter from outside the oral cavity or are completely contained within it. Some of the key salivary glands are the parotids, mandibulars, and sublinguals. A parotid gland is located on each side of the head. It sits within a nest of fascia, ventral to the pinna. It opens into the oral cavity from the area of the maxilla, around the teeth called premolars.

The mandibular glands open onto the ventral mouth. The sublingual glands are rostral to the mandibular glands and have numerous small ducts. Certain disease states can cause the salivary glands to become inflamed. If indicated, removal of some of these glands can be accomplished. However, this is done with great difficulty due to their size and location within other important areas of the oral cavity.

The mucosal tissue that contains the teeth is referred to as the gingiva. Their color can be a major indicator of disease states. A pale pink or white color is often associated with anemia. A blue tinge may indicate cyanosis, a lack of sufficient oxygen within the bloodstream. Yellow can be an indication of hepatic disease. A brown, muddy color may reflect methemoglobinemia, associated with carbon monoxide poisoning. In addition, a tacky (sticky), dry condition of the gingiva reflects dehydration. Palpation of the gingiva should be a part of any physical examination.

The teeth are variable in number among species (see Figure 9.2). The upper set of teeth is referred to as the maxillary arcade, and the lower teeth the mandibular arcade. The names of the

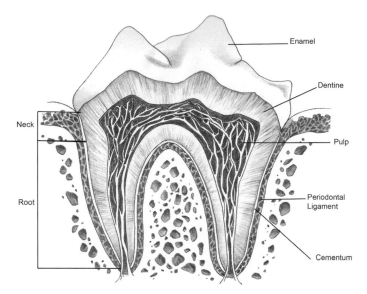

Figure 9.3   Parts of the tooth. The crown is covered by enamel. The bulk of the tooth consists of dentine. The pulp cavity contains vessels and nerves. The neck of the tooth intersects with gingiva. Each of the two roots is seated in the alveolus, which is the socket in the bone the tooth sits in.

teeth are characterized by their location and shape. The rostral-most, rectangular teeth are referred to as incisors. Caudal to them are longer, cone-shaped teeth referred to as the canine teeth. Caudal to them are the premolar teeth, which often have a sharp or irregular dorsal surface. The caudal-most teeth are the molars.

In order to identify the teeth, a formula is utilized. The number of each type of tooth is listed from rostral to caudal, with the maxillary teeth above the mandibular teeth, separated by a line. The formula represents half of the arcade. An adult dog's formula is 3142/3143. This indicates that on each side of the maxilla, there are three incisors, one canine, four premolars, and two molars. Note that each mandibular section includes one additional molar. The formula for the adult cat is 3131/3121. The teeth are identified by a letter and a number, or just a number. For example, I2 refers to the second incisor (counting from the midline). The other abbreviations are C, PM, and M. A method of assigning numbers to each tooth is the Triadan system, used in dental settings. See Figure 21.1 for an illustration of this numbering pattern.

As in primates, there are deciduous ("baby") teeth, which are ejected as the permanent ("adult") teeth grow in. It is useful to reassure a client that the deciduous teeth are rarely found once they come out, and that there should not be any concern if these teeth are "missing." Unexplained loss of the adult tooth, particularly in a younger animal, warrants a visit to the clinic, however.

The tooth itself is called the dens (see Figure 9.3). It is composed of a number of parts. The crown is the visible part and is covered by a hard material called enamel. The root of the tooth, which should be completely embedded within the gingiva, is covered by a different material called cementum. Cementum and enamel cover a substance called dentin, which makes up the bulk of the tooth. Between the crown and the root, there is a slight indentation called the neck of the tooth.

The socket in which each tooth sits is called the alveolus. The gingiva should extend up to the neck of the tooth. Exposure of the neck and root of the tooth is an indication of dental disease. At the very center of the tooth is a connective tissue called pulp. The nerve supplying each tooth runs through this area. The roots of the teeth are eventually embedded in the jaw.

The various teeth have different functions, which will be discussed in Chapter 21. For now, note that the different shapes facilitate their function. The incisors have a single root (prong), as do the canines. The root of the canine is particularly long, anchoring this large tooth securely. Premolars have two roots, as do molars. In cats, the third maxillary premolar and first mandibular molar are known as the carnassial teeth; in dogs, it is the fourth maxillary premolar and the first mandibular molar that are the carnassial teeth. These teeth have three roots and are particularly difficult to extract.

The pharynx and the esophagus

The vestibule of the oral cavity opens into a large space called the pharynx (essentially, the throat). Ingesta are conducted through the pharynx into the esophagus, which connects with the stomach. The area immediately caudal to the vestibule is referred to as the oropharynx. It merges with the nasopharynx, which is caudal to the nasal passages. Thus, the pharynx carries both air and food (and whatever else the animal has eaten; those familiar with Labrador retrievers know them as a breed that will try to swallow just about anything, including rocks). The pharynx narrows as it approaches the larynx, where it is referred to as the laryngopharynx. Food is then directed into the esophagus.

The cervical part of the esophagus courses through the neck of the animal. It is crucial to remember that the esophagus runs to the left of the trachea (the animal's left) in this area. When placing an esophageal feeding tube, the animal should be in right lateral recumbency so that the left side, and thus the esophagus, is available.

The section of the esophagus from the thoracic inlet to the diaphragm is known as the thoracic esophagus. The esophagus passes through an opening in the diaphragm called the esophageal hiatus as it travels toward the stomach. The short section from the diaphragm to the stomach is referred to as the abdominal esophagus. Note that these divisions represent sections of the same long tube and are used for convenience in description rather than for reasons of microanatomy.

The esophagus is composed of several layers. The outer layer, the serosa, is composed of connective tissue. There is a muscular layer as well, and the luminal layer is mucosal tissue. There are two layers of muscle tissue, one longitudinal and one circular. Even within small animal species, there are structural differences. In dogs, the esophagus is lined by striated muscle throughout its length. In cats, the distal (caudal) section of the esophagus is smooth muscle. The distal esophageal sphincter is called the cardiac sphincter.

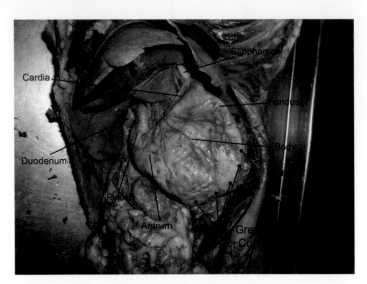

Box 9.1   Abdominal quadrants

The abdomen is divided into four quadrants. The divisions are right cranial, right caudal, left cranial, and left caudal. Elements within each division may be easier to visualize this way.

Right cranial quadrant: pancreas, part of the liver
Right caudal quadrant: descending duodenum, cecum
Left cranial quadrant: fundus and body of stomach, left lobes of the liver
Left caudal quadrant: descending colon

Figure 9.4   Sections of the stomach. The animal's head is toward the top of the picture. The greater curvature anchors the omentum, which is a fatty "blanket" that covers the viscera along their ventral surfaces.

Once the esophagus passes the diaphragm, it has entered the abdominal cavity. The esophagus itself enters the stomach. Further discussion of the abdomen is warranted here. The abdominal cavity is the space caudal to the diaphragm, extending to the pubic brim (pelvic cavity). It is the largest of the body cavities. It is further divided into two sections: the peritoneal space and the retroperitoneum. The peritoneum is a membranous sac, within which are most of the visceral organs. The sac itself, composed of connective tissue, also covers the serosal surface of many of the organs. The accumulation of fluid within the peritoneal space is referred to as ascites and is an indication of severe disease states such as cardiac or hepatic dysfunction, or the viral disease feline infectious peritonitis (FIP). The retroperitoneum, an area in the caudal abdominal cavity, is the space between the peritoneum and the body wall. It contains lymph nodes, the kidneys, the ureters, and parts of the reproductive tract.

Within the peritoneum are folds of connective tissue that suspend the small and large intestines from the body wall. This is referred to as the mesentery and carries blood vessels and lymphatic vessels to and from the digestive tract. They arise from a thick base, called the root of the mesentery, present in the dorsal part of the cavity.

For the purpose of description, the abdomen is divided into quadrants (Box 9.1). A clue toward analyzing the situation presented at the beginning of this chapter lies in this system of locating organs. The area of the caudal abdomen just medial to the pelvic limbs is referred to as the inguinal area.

The stomach

The structure of the stomach is particularly species specific (see Figures 9.4 and 9.5). In dogs and cats, which are omnivores and carnivores, respectively, the high level of concentration of nutrients in their food allows stomach structure to be relatively simple. The superficial layer, the serosa, is connective tissue. Deep to this is a layer of smooth muscle. Next is a layer including elastic fibers, nerves, and blood and lymphatic vessels. The luminal surface is composed of epithelium and mucosa, as well as a large number of glands.

The elastic fibers corrugate to form rugae (ridges). The fuller the stomach is, the less prominent they are. A stomach relatively

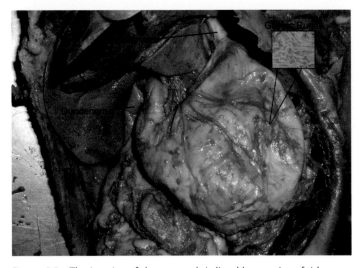

Figure 9.5   The interior of the stomach is lined by a series of ridges called rugae. These can expand and help increase the surface area of the stomach during digestion. On the other hand, the rugae of the hard palate are fixed in position.

empty of ingesta will have the appearance of a star apple on ultrasonography. Rugae increase the surface area of the digestive tissue.

The named areas of the stomach vary in shape. The cardia is a short section where the esophagus enters. The tubelike section caudal to it is the fundus. This opens into a large cavity running on a transverse axis across the cranial abdomen, called the body of the stomach. Continuing caudolaterally is a short, narrower section called the pyloric antrum. Lateroventral to this is the pyloris, a short canal that contains the pyloric sphincter. This smooth muscle sphincter opens when food is ready to travel through it.

The cranial curve of the body of the stomach is known as the lesser curvature. It is linked by connective tissue to the liver. The longer, bowl-shaped, caudal border is known as the greater curvature of the stomach. Attached to the greater curvature of the stomach is a large sheet of fat and connective tissue called the omentum. It has a lacy appearance and covers the ventral surface of the peritoneal cavity like a curtain. Within the omentum is the gastrosplenic ligament, providing the spleen with an anchor to the stomach. The majority of the omentum is superfluous and is often used as graft tissue; that is, a section of omentum can be excised and placed into a gap to form a soft-tissue bridge when tissue is damaged.

The major blood supply of the stomach is the celiac artery. Most of the veins of the stomach join the portal vein. There are many lymphatic glands and vessels. Innervation is both sympathetic and parasympathetic.

The intestines

The pyloric sphincter is the gateway to the small intestine. In order of the passage of nutrients, the sections are the duodenum, jejunum, and ileum (see Figures 9.6 and 9.7). The pancreas, an organ with both endocrine and exocrine functions, runs along the medial surface of the duodenum. Its exocrine functions, those that relate to sending out enzymes or other chemical messengers, include releasing digestive enzymes into the intestinal tract. In dogs and cats, there is a small section of vestigial (no longer physiologically necessary) tissue called the cecum, marking the border between the small and large intestines. In contrast, the cecum is well developed and crucial to digestion in species such as rodents, rabbits, and equines. The tissue of the small intestine has several layers, also called tunics. They include

a serosal layer, a layer of muscle and elastic tissue, and a layer of epithelial tissue.

Exiting the ileum, the tube that is the intestine becomes the colon. At its caudal end, it widens into a chamber called the rectum. Material exits the body at the anus, a sphincter with smooth and striated muscle components.

The intestines are often referred to as the gut. In the carnivore, it is relatively short—approximately three to four times the length of the trunk. In comparison, the gut is 25 times the length of the trunk in sheep.

The duodenum is a relatively short section forming a "J" shape. The descending limb heads toward the right kidney, with the ascending limb curving around to point toward the stomach. The curve itself is the medial section between them. Contained in the descending limb are the major and minor papillae (in the dog; there is only one in the cat). These openings accommodate the bile duct and the pancreatic duct. In some animals, there are actually two pancreatic ducts. On careful examination of the luminal surface of the duodenum, you may see the papillae.

The pancreas is in the dorsal abdomen and runs alongside the medial surface of the descending limb of the duodenum. Its larger amount of tissue is devoted to the production of digestive enzymes. In life, it has a pink, cobblestone appearance. It is supplied by the celiac and mesenteric arteries and drains to the portal vein. As is true for most of the gastrointestinal (GI) tract, there is sympathetic and parasympathetic innervation. Note that the pancreas has endocrine tissue as well; one of the crucial hormones it produces is insulin. When we discuss endocrine

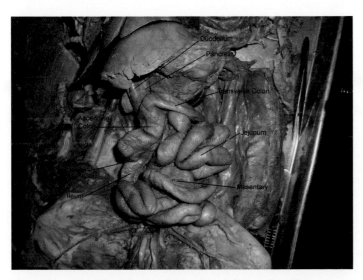

Figure 9.6   Sections of the small intestine and the colon. The descending colon continues caudally from the transverse colon and is underneath the jejunum in this picture. The three sections of the colon (ascending, transverse, and descending) are referred to as the large intestine. Note that in the living animal, the positions of the parts of the intestinal tract change slightly as they move.

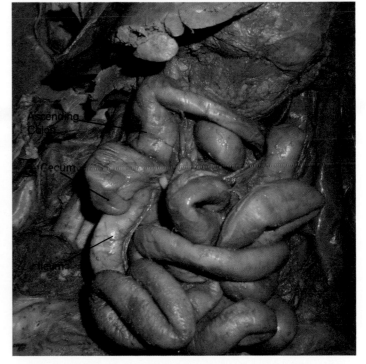

Figure 9.7   The ileum enters the cecum, which in dogs and cats is vestigial, as the ingesta continue toward the colon.

physiology, we will describe the function of this hormone; abnormalities of its production or function are involved in a common metabolic disease, diabetes mellitus.

From the ascending duodenum, the small intestine coils numerous times. The jejunum and ileum are suspended from the mesentery and are not anchored to any other part of the abdomen. When serial radiographs are taken, the small intestine will change its position as it contracts and expands these coils. A lack of change over a number of hours can help verify intestinal stasis, known as ileus; this is a potentially fatal condition wherein the intestines no longer contract and expand as they usually do. The ileum turns toward the right as it runs toward the cecum. The ileocolic junction denotes this connection.

The border between the jejunum and the ileum is merely a functional one. On gross visual inspection, it is hard to point to the spot where the change occurs. This can only be determined on histologic examination (looking at microscopic sections from a biopsy sample).

In dogs, the cecum connects to the ascending colon. The cecum is a blind alley that forms a slight spiral. A condition called intussusception occurs when part of the intestine telescopes into another. Ileocecal intussusception is a common type of intussusception in dogs and is readily surgically cured as long as it is treated quickly.

The ascending colon is relatively short in the carnivore. The transverse colon travels from the right toward the stomach, in an area between the stomach and the small intestine. Again, note that the intestine is mobile so that the exact positioning of the transverse colon will vary. The longest part of the colon is the descending limb. It runs along the left flank, turns slightly medially at the pelvic cavity, and widens to become the rectum. The distal descending colon exits the peritoneum to course in the retroperitoneum. The rectum is dorsal to the reproductive organs. It has a connective tissue attachment to the vagina (to the urethra in the male).

In a ventrolateral position between the internal and external anal sphincters are the anal sacs. There is one on each side of the anus, and their opening can be seen from the outside of the animal. These glands are compressed at defecation. They are sebaceous glands whose viscous fluid has a strong odor. This fluid can be discharged under stress. Skunks can voluntarily expel this fluid, which is an effective defense mechanism. The anal glands of dogs and cats can become clogged and may need to be manually expressed during physical examinations in the clinic. Animals that "scoot" (rub their perineum along the floor while moving forward) often have impacted anal glands.

The blood supply of the intestines originates mostly from the cranial and caudal mesenteric arteries; the proximal duodenum is supplied by the celiac artery and the caudal rectum by the internal pudendal artery. Many of the veins eventually empty into the portal vein. There is a tremendous amount of lymphatic drainage, most of which goes to the thoracic duct. There are many lymph nodes within the mesentery. Notice that the vessels are present in very large numbers within the mesentery and that each section of the intestine gets blood from a variety of arteries. This is the basis of collateral circulation, which refers to redun-

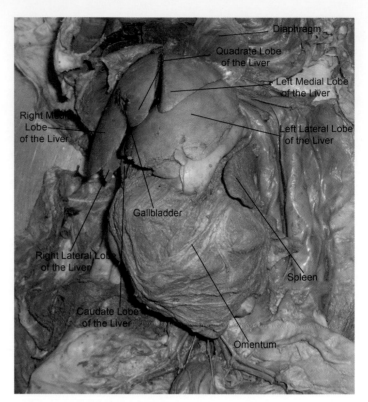

Figure 9.8 The lobes of the liver.

dancy in the blood supply. If one or even a few of these vessels are damaged or surgically interrupted, the intestine still has a sufficient number of circulatory vessels. Sympathetic and parasympathetic innervation is present.

The liver

The liver has a number of important functions. One of its major roles is as part of the digestive process. It is located caudal to the diaphragm, stretching from the midline toward the animal's right (see Figure 9.8). In addition to contributing to the metabolism of nutrients, it aids in the production of bile. Blood containing absorbed nutrients travels from the GI tract via the portal circulatory system, is processed by the liver, and then is either released to the general circulation or back to the GI tract.

The mammalian liver has distinct lobes. In dogs and cats, they are the left lateral, left medial, right lateral, right medial, quadrate, and caudate lobes. The gallbladder lies between the quadrate and right medial lobes. The liver's serosal surface has fossae (concavities) in which the stomach and the right kidney sit. There are also grooves that accommodate the caudal vena cava and the esophagus. The falciform ligament, the remnant of an embryonic vessel, attaches the liver to the diaphragm.

The circulation to and from the liver routes material from and to the digestive tract, as well as filtering material to the rest of the peripheral circulation. Arterial inputs include the hepatic and celiac arteries, and the major vein is the portal vein. The liver is connected by a large duct to the gallbladder and by

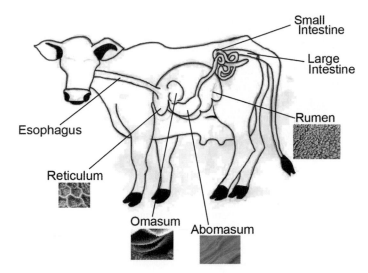

Figure 9.9   Features of the bovine digestive tract.

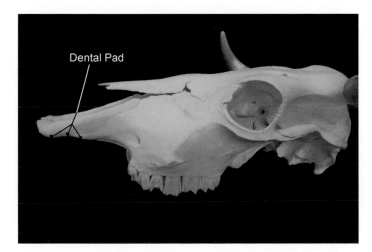

Figure 9.10   The dental pad is not actually pictured here; the lines point to where it would be. In the living animal, it forms the area where the maxillary incisor teeth would be and allows the crushing movement necessary to process grasses and fibers.

a smaller duct to the duodenum. Innervation is sympathetic and parasympathetic.

Species variation

The lips of ruminants, and equines to an even larger extent, are much thicker and more mobile than in dogs and cats. This assists in the prehension of food. These areas are well innervated. The release of endorphins that occur when a twitch is wound around the lips of a horse relies in part on the large number of nerve endings that are present.

The dentition of the ruminant is unique (see Figure 9.10). There are no maxillary incisors. In their place, there is a thick mass of tissue called a dental pad. This allows the

tough, fibrous material they eat to be ground against the pad's flat surface.

Equines and lagomorphs (rabbits) have a great deal in common from a physiological standpoint. Unlike mammals, the majority of their food is digested in the cecum (as opposed to the stomach). Thus, the cecum is relatively much larger, and the stomach much smaller, than in dogs and cats. As their diet has almost no fat, equines do not require bile for digestion. Rats, equines, and lamoids do not have a gallbladder.

A most striking adaptation to diet is present in ruminants (see Figure 9.9). Ruminants have a four-chambered stomach, which receives the crushed food materials from the oral cavity. The cranial-most part of the stomach is the reticulum. Its lining contains many small compartments and may be familiar as the food item tripe. This cavity lies directly caudal to the heart. In foraging for food, ruminants will occasionally take in nails, fence wire, and other sharp items. They can actually penetrate the reticulum and perforate the heart. The condition, formally known as traumatic reticulopericarditis and informally known as "hardware disease," is fairly common. The treatment for this is to have the animal swallow a magnet, which prevents any future metal from migrating outside the reticulum.

Caudal to the reticulum is the largest chamber, the rumen (the root word of the species designation, ruminant). The next chamber is the omasum, and the last is the abomasum. This latter section is closest to the mammalian stomach in structure and function.

In some ruminants, there is a short section of intestine that ends in a descending colon. In goats, the colon has a spiral shape.

The equine colon is particularly long and consists of a tube that folds over on itself, then travels to the other side of the animal and folds over on itself again. There are smaller folds called haustra along some of the length of the colon. They can be palpated on rectal exam and help the examiner pinpoint his/her location within the cavity.

Avians have a quite different system. They have a beak rather than lips and do not have teeth. As food enters the oral cavity, it is often stored in a space called the crop, in the ventral neck. Food travels along the esophagus to the stomach, which has two chambers, the ventriculus and the proventriculus. Material is then discharged via the cloaca, a chamber that is shared with the reproductive tract (see Figure 9.11).

Clinical case resolution: Dog with diarrhea and pain

The case described at the beginning of the chapter presents data consistent with pancreatitis. One of the clues to this is the pain located in the right cranial quadrant of the abdomen, the location of the pancreas. Copious, watery diarrhea is associated with small rather than large intestinal disease. As the pancreas and duodenum run together, it is very common for inflammation in one of those areas to affect the other.

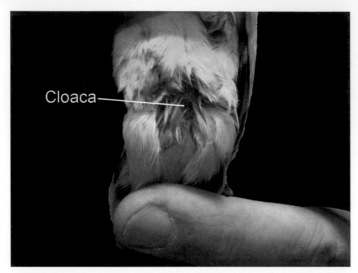

Figure 9.11   The cloaca is the common exit from the avian body for the digestive, urinary, and reproductive tracts.

Review questions

1 What structure marks the caudal extent of the oral vestibule?
2 Which has more teeth under normal circumstances, a cat or a dog?
3 The fundus and body of the stomach lie in which quadrant of the abdomen?
4 Which segment of the small intestine is directly distal to the pyloric sphincter?
5 The three parts of the colon, or large intestine, are _____.
6 Inflammation of the pancreas is associated with inflammation of the small intestine because _____.
7 What are the four parts of the bovine stomach?
8 Rabbits and horses do most of their digestion in the _____.

Chapter **10** Anatomy of the Endocrine System

Clinical case: Thirsty cat with weight loss

A client brings a 10-year-old cat into the clinic. The cat has been drinking a great deal of water and has been losing weight. In fact, she is losing weight even though her appetite has increased. In palpating her ventral neck, you feel an enlarged area on either side of the trachea, caudal to the larynx. The interpretation of these findings will be explained as this chapter continues.

Introduction

The endocrine system is largely responsible for the metabolism of cats and dogs. Its malfunction is the cause of a wide variety of common chronic diseases. We will discuss the physiology of the system in detail in Chapter 22. Its systemic anatomy is somewhat unusual in that it is a single system which has components spread throughout the body.

The constituents of the endocrine system are referred to as glands. Unlike other glands (e.g., those of the skin), they do not have ducts that conduct their products to other areas or organs. Their products are carried through the body as a result of close contact between the endocrine gland and the bloodstream. Therefore, in addition to rich neural innervations, they are well vascularized.

The hypothalamus and the pituitary

There are a number of sites throughout the central nervous system that play a role in the management of endocrine products (hormones). The primary ones are in the area of the hypothalamus, from which source neural signals travel through a narrow stalk to the pituitary gland. The latter occupies a fossa on the ventral surface of the brain, called the sella turcica, and depends from it.

The monitoring sensors within the hypothalamus respond to exterior stimuli and send neural impulses by way of the pituitary gland (also known as the hypophysis). The pituitary is ellipsoid in shape and dark in color. Rostral and caudal to it is the cavernous sinus of the brain. It sits in the sella turcica ("Turkish saddle"), a structure on the ventral surface of the braincase. The pituitary has three lobes, the anterior, intermediate, and posterior. This is a rare example of the use of the terms anterior and posterior instead of cranial and caudal. Each of these lobes produces or stimulates the production of particular hormones. The variety of messenger chemicals produced earned the pituitary the title of the "master gland."

Anatomy and Physiology for Veterinary Technicians and Nurses: A Clinical Approach, First Edition. Robin Sturtz and Lori Asprea.
© 2012 John Wiley & Sons, Inc. Published 2012 by John Wiley & Sons, Inc.

Another gland in this area is the pineal gland. (Its name comes from the root word for "pineapple," which it is said to resemble.) It is in the area of the third ventricle of the brain. It is also known as the epiphysis and will not be readily identifiable on necropsy. In reptiles, some breeds have a pineal gland that resides on the dorsal brain and actually receives sunlight directly from the outside. This is useful for animals that govern their metabolism using hours of daylight to restrict or increase activity. In the equine, it can also influence the transition out of anestrus to seasonal estrous cycles; estrus ("heat") will be discussed in Chapter 24.

The peripheral endocrine system

Glands that function only in producing and/or managing the production of hormones are known as primary endocrine glands. One of the major primary endocrine glands is the thyroid gland. It is a C-shaped gland that wraps around the trachea from the lateral to the dorsal surface and then to the other lateral surface. Depending on the species, the dorsal connection can be very thin or the same width as the rest of the gland. The thyroid is dark red in color and has a connective tissue covering. It is considered to consist of two lobes (see Figure 10.1).

Under normal conditions, it should not be easily palpable in the dog and cat. During physical exam, running the fingers along either side of the trachea may yield the sensation of a swelling that interrupts the smooth flow of the palpation. This is known as "thyroid slip" and is associated with enlargement of the thyroid gland. This enlargement is associated with hyperthyroidism, a condition common in older cats that causes increased appetite and weight loss.

In viewing the thyroid gland on dissection, one may observe a small lump on the surface of the thyroid or partially embedded

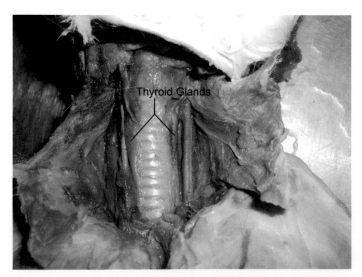

Figure 10.1   The thyroid glands viewed with the animal in dorsal recumbency. Note that they do not cover the ventral surface of the trachea. The cartilaginous rings that support the trachea are clearly visible as the white bands that wrap horizontally around the trachea.

within it. There is one on each side, and they are referred to as the parathyroid glands. They are pale in color. As will be seen later, they have a great deal to do with calcium and phosphorus balance within the body. One reason that thyroidectomy is rarely employed as a treatment for hyperthyroidism is that it is difficult to avoid disrupting the parathyroid glands in the process. (Another reason for possible complication following this surgery is that ectopic thyroid is occasionally present, which will continue to function even if the primary gland is removed.)

Another primary endocrine gland is the adrenal gland. The adrenal gland is a small, pinkish, smooth structure slightly cranial or craniomedial to the kidney (see Figure 10.2). There is one on each side of the body. The adrenals are firm and solid and have two sections, a medulla and a cortex. This gland will often be surrounded by fat, so careful displacement of the perirenal fat layer is important. Running on the ventral surface of the adrenal gland are the thoracolumbar vein and artery.

The adrenal gland has bands of tissue, each of which produces discrete hormones (Figure 10.3). The adrenal cortex produces glucocorticoids, mineralocorticoids, and reproductive hormones. The adrenal medulla, deep to the cortex and more or less in the center of the gland, produces important neurotransmitters.

Secondary endocrine glands are areas manufacturing hormones that are within organs or tissue that have nonendocrine features. The best known of these is the endocrine tissue within the pancreas. The endocrine areas of the pancreas are called the islets of Langerhans.

These areas are involved in the production of insulin, among other hormones. The function of the alpha and beta cells of the islets will be discussed later. Bear in mind that these structures are microscopic. Gross inspection of the pancreas on dissection will not yield an appreciable difference in structure between the endocrine and nonendocrine tissues within the pancreas.

Because the pancreas has a connection to the duodenum for the transfer of digestive enzymes, inflammatory bowel disease can be associated with pancreatitis. Pancreatitis, in turn, can be associated with inflammation of the endocrine sections as well, which is why diabetes mellitus (an insulin-based disorder) can be associated with chronic enteritis and/or pancreatitis.

Parts of the reproductive system have secondary endocrine tissue. These include the testes, ovaries, and the placenta. Small amounts of endocrine tissue are also found within the small intestine, liver, and thymus. There are even small amounts of endocrine tissue in the heart. Again, none of this endocrine material is macroscopic.

Another part of the secondary endocrine system is the nephron, particularly the area around the glomerulus. A small number of endocrine cells within the nephron produce a hormone called erythropoietin. This chemical messenger is vital in stimulating the bone marrow to produce red blood cells and is one of the reasons that we associate chronic kidney disease in its more severe states with anemia. Without those endocrine cells, the bone marrow no longer produces sufficient red blood cells.

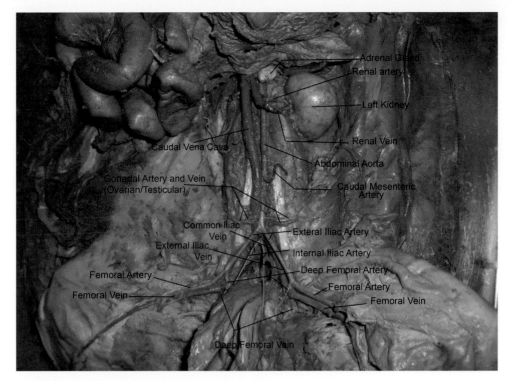

Figure 10.2　The adrenal gland (this photograph also appears in Chapter 8).

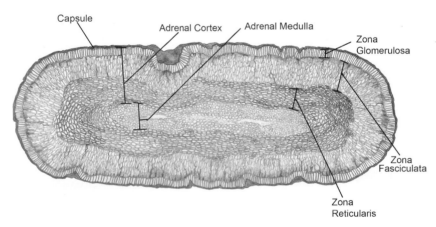

Figure 10.3　Drawing of sagittal section of adrenal gland. Note the capsule surrounding the gland, the three layers of the cortex (some people use the mnemonic device GFR to remember their names), and irregular shape and spacing of the cells of the medulla.

Clinical case resolution: Thirsty cat with weight loss

Based on the information provided at the beginning of the chapter, it is most likely that the cat is suffering from hyperthyroidism. Hyperthyroidism, along with diabetes mellitus, is the most common metabolic diseases in older cats. It is readily treated in most cases. Hypothyroidism is known in cats but is rare. The reverse is true in dogs; hypothyroidism is fairly common, but hyperthyroidism is rare. A patient with hyperthyroidism usually has a strong appetite and drinks a great deal, and loses significant weight. This relates to the thyroid's function as a regulator of the speed of metabolism. (Note, however, that these findings are also noted in other diseases.) The swelling noted in the neck is the enlarged thyroid gland.

Review questions

1 What is contained in the sella turcica?
2 What party of the body is the thyroid gland located in?
3 What does the pineal gland do?
4 What is the location of the adrenal glands?
5 Where are the insulin-producing cells located? Does this organ have any nonendocrine functions? What are they?

Chapter **11** Respiratory Anatomy

Clinical case: Dyspneic dog

At 1:00 am, an emergency clinic receives a dog that is dyspneic. There is a history of several days of increased respiratory effort and exercise intolerance. The dog, a German Shepherd, has a mucoid nasal discharge. The family lives in the Four Corners area of the southwestern United States and often goes into a local area for photography and hiking. The dog comes along on many of these outings. They have not had any of these trips in at least several weeks.

Introduction

The respiratory system begins at the nose in most terrestrial animals. In dogs and cats, the nose is merged into the muzzle. Its mucocutaneous border, where skin transitions into mucous membrane, is often the site of skin diseases associated with autoimmune disorders, so its superficial surface always requires close inspection on physical exam. The nose provides not only a conduit for the passage of air but is involved in olfaction. It also warms and humidifies air, reducing irritation to the tissues of the upper respiratory system. It is also noteworthy that the tear ducts empty into the nostrils; one way that we can assess the patency of the tear duct is to introduce saline into the duct and see if it runs out the nose.

Entry into the respiratory system

The external opening into the nasal passage is known as the nostril. The nostrils are also referred to as nares, and the terms are essentially interchangeable. The outer walls of the nostrils are made of cartilage. The lateral surfaces of these walls are referred to as nasal alae (from the Latin root meaning "wings"). The exterior central groove visible between the nares is referred to as the nasal philtrum. The flat area between the nostrils (containing the philtrum) is the nasal planum.

The short tunnel at the entrance to the nasal passage is called the nasal vestibule. It narrows slightly as it runs caudally on each side; each passage is separated by a cartilaginous wall called the nasal septum, which runs medially and caudally. The wall becomes bone by the time it reaches the level of the ethmoid bone.

The lining of the interior surface of the nasal passages is mucous membrane, with many ciliated cells. Some of this tissue

Anatomy and Physiology for Veterinary Technicians and Nurses: A Clinical Approach, First Edition. Robin Sturtz and Lori Asprea.
© 2012 John Wiley & Sons, Inc. Published 2012 by John Wiley & Sons, Inc.

is erectile; this function is particularly triggered in cases of inflammation.

As the cartilaginous section ends, there is a bony wall composed of shell-like scrollwork called the concha, or nasal turbinates. The concha is divided into three major openings, called the dorsal, middle, and ventral meatus, respectively. As air passes through the dorsal meatus, it flows over olfactory mucosa. Air that continues via the middle meatus directs air to the pharynx.

The frontal sinus is dorsal to the ethmoid area; the maxillary sinus is deep and ventral to the eye. Both are lined by mucous membrane that is continuous with that of the nasal mucosa. This is how inflammation travels into the sinus. Note that the respiratory mucosa is involved in the pathway to the olfactory system as well; it is for this reason that diminished sense of smell often accompanies upper respiratory inflammation. This factor is a particular issue in cats, which depend to a great extent on their sense of smell as a stimulus to ingestion.

As air continues ventrally from the nasal passage, it passes through the oropharynx, which includes the caudal section of the oral cavity and the dorsal section of the pharynx. As the air continues caudally, it arrives at the larynx, which is the boundary between the pharynx and the trachea.

The larynx

The cranial part of the larynx has connections to the hyoid apparatus (the chain of small bones running from the skull and connecting with the larynx and the base of the tongue), which is why the larynx moves when the animal swallows. A stalk of cartilage in the shape of a leaf is attached to the cranial larynx and is referred to as the epiglottis. The epiglottis closes over the laryngeal opening when the animal swallows so that liquid and solid materials go into the esophagus instead of the trachea and then the lungs.

The larynx itself is composed of a series of cartilages. The largest is the cranial-most, and is called the thyroid cartilage. It forms the palpable sides, and the ventral surface, of the larynx. The rostral part of it comes to a point that, in humans, is referred to as the "Adam's apple."

The name of the next cartilage in the series, the cricoid cartilage, comes from the Latin root for a signet ring, which it resembles. It is caudodorsal to and articulated with the thyroid cartilage. The third structure is actually a pair of somewhat triangular cartilages that sit inside the cricoid cartilage and rock back and forth. They provide the attachment for the vocal folds, and the mobility of the cartilages allows for the vibration of the folds. These are called the arytenoid cartilages.

The opening between the vocal folds is known as the glottis. It is lined by epithelium and a thick layer of mucous membrane. When the glottis is open, then air passes through into or out of the trachea. Air passing on its way out causes the vocal folds to vibrate, which is part of how the animal makes sound. Again, this has tremendous import from a clinical standpoint; in placing an endotracheal tube, it must be placed between the vocal folds, through the glottis, in order for air to reach the lungs.

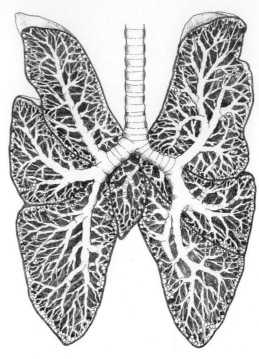

Figure 11.1   The trachea (center, top), which branches into smaller and smaller airways, from the main bronchi to bronchioles. The area between the lungs is referred to as the mediastinum.

The trachea and lungs

The continuation of the airway past the larynx is the trachea. It is a fibrous tube marked by a series of cartilaginous rings. These rings are incomplete in the dog and cat in that the dorsal surface is composed of fibrous tissue rather than cartilage. The inner lining of the trachea consists of ciliated cells, with the middle and outer linings made of fibrous material. In performing a tracheotomy, the goal is to surgically form an opening in between the rings.

The trachea enters the thorax at the mediastinum, the medial space between the lung lobes (see Figure 11.1). Dorsal to the heart, the trachea branches into the two main bronchi. This spot is considered to be the division between the upper and lower respiratory tracts. Each main bronchus maintains the rings as it enters each side of the lung, after which the rings disappear.

As the bronchus enters the lobes of the lung, it divides into a series of smaller and smaller branches. The smallest are known as bronchioles. At their terminus, they become a series of small sacs known as alveoli. Their function is crucial to respiration, which will be discussed in Chapter 23.

The pleura consists of two layers of serosal material; the parietal pleura lines the interior of the thoracic cavity, and the visceral pleura lines the lungs themselves. There is a small amount of viscous material in between the layers, which lubricates the tissues and helps maintain negative pressure within the chest cavity. The concepts of pleural effusion and pleuritis, then, refer not to the lung tissues themselves but to the surrounding layers.

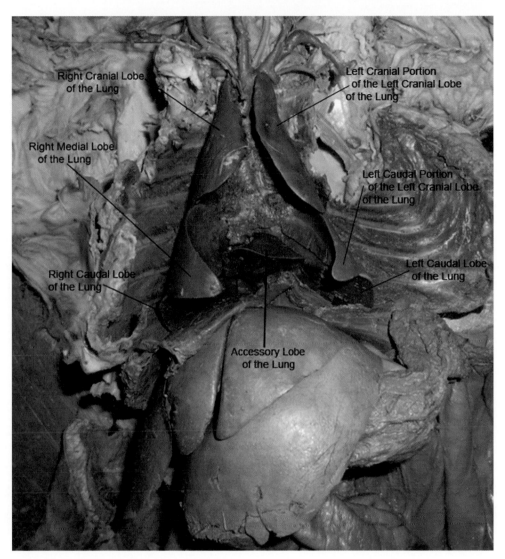

Figure 11.2   Lobes of the lung.

The visceral pleura folds around the cranial part of the lungs, near the branching of the main bronchi. While the main bronchi cannot be seen on radiography, the borders of the mediastinal space are visible on radiography. The ability to see it is important in diagnosing many disease conditions. The area where the main bronchi diverge is the only place at which the lungs are anchored to the body; the rest of the lungs are free-floating within the thoracic cavity.

Pulmonary tissue itself is composed of elastic, spongy material. In the moments after birth, the lungs fill with air. One way to determine if a newborn that is dead has passed away before or after birth is to take a sample of lung tissue and see if it floats. Before birth, it will not have any air in it yet, so the tissue will sink in water. If the newborn died after birth, when the lung had filled with air, the tissue will float.

The number of lobes (sections) the lung has varies greatly by species, as does their outside appearance. In dogs and cats, there are three lobes on the left and four on the right (see Figure 11.2).

On the left, there are the cranial, middle, and caudal lobes. Note that some people refer to these lobes as the cranial part of the cranial lobe and the caudal part of the cranial lobe. They are followed by the left caudal lobe. On the right, there are cranial, middle, and caudal lobes, as well as a smaller section called the accessory lobe. The accessory lobe is in a caudodorsal position and fits into a fold in the parietal pleura. In dogs and cats, the connective tissue that makes up the lungs has small thickened fibers that give the lungs their "cobblestone" appearance.

The function of the system is dependent on each of its parts, from the opening of the nostrils to the air exchange at the surface of the alveoli. The distinction between the upper and lower respiratory systems is particularly important from a clinical standpoint. For example, the presence of crackling sounds when ausculting the thorax is associated with lower rather than upper respiratory disease.

The cranial-most part of the lung is referred to as the apex and the caudal part as the base. The diaphragm, a thick fibrous tissue that spans the width of the thorax, is at the base of the thorax. There are openings for the aorta and the veins, called the aortal hiatus, and the esophagus, called the esophageal hiatus. A hiatal hernia is an abnormal opening or tear in the diaphragm; diaphragmatic hernia can be congenital or caused by trauma and can actually allow parts of the abdominal organs to be pulled up into the thorax.

Box 11.1   Some clinical considerations

The tissue on the ventral surface of the lung lobes is rather thin. In auscultation, lateral and ventral sites will yield better information regarding lung sounds.

There are lymph nodes situated throughout the thorax. Enlargement of those just dorsal to the heart and dorsal to the third sternebra will give an abnormal appearance on radiography of the thorax and may cause the mediastinum to appear wide on ventrodorsal view.

The smaller airways should not be visible on radiography. If they are, they are most likely inflamed. The bronchial arteries, on the other hand, are often visible.

Species differentiation

The nasal passage in the nose of the horse has a small diverticulum, or blind alley. Caution needs to be exercised when placing a feeding tube into the nose. The tube could inadvertently be guided into the diverticulum, which would not be helpful.

The pig has a bony plate in the area of the canine/feline philtrum. This is known as the rostral plate.

The horse has a third main bronchus, on the right side of the mediastinum.

The pig has a highly lobulated appearance to the lungs, the surface of which appear as pebbles. The lungs of the horse are smooth.

The lungs of the avian are rather small and do not expand in the process of inhalation and exhalation. The gas exchange of respiration takes place in the lung. On the other hand, there are air sacs, which look like Bubble Wrap, which are spread throughout the thorax and abdomen and do the actual expanding and contraction. This will be discussed further in Chapter 23.

Clinical case resolution: Dyspneic dog

The dog is given a series of tests, including radiography of the head and chest and culture of the nasal discharge. While treatment is ongoing, the culture reveals the presence of a fungus, aspergillus. It is most likely that the dog inhaled the spores while on one of the family's outings. Treatment with an antifungal medication effects a complete cure.

Review questions

1 What is the tissue lining the inside of the thoracic cavity?
2 What are the rings of the trachea made of?
3 What is the groove between the nostrils on the outside of the nose called?
4 How many lobes of the lungs do dogs and cats have?
5 What is the opening between the vocal folds called?

Chapter **12** Reproductive Anatomy

Clinical case: Canine orchiectomy

A dog is brought into the clinic for orchiectomy. The scrotum on one side appears to be empty on palpation (i.e., does not have a testicle within it). The other side has a normal testicle, which is removed without incident. In this cryptorchid animal, where would one start looking for the ectopic testicle?

Introduction

The anatomy of the reproductive system also varies remarkably in structure across mammalian species. In addition, the system in reptiles and fish is quite different from that in mammals. The reproductive system actually changes shape and size during adulthood as well as in youth, under certain neural and endocrine influences. It is particularly affected by age-related factors, both at the beginning and the end of life (Box 12.1).

The female

The ovary is the cranial-most part of the system. It is solid and ellipsoid, and within a given breed is of a constant size regardless

of body weight. There is significant breed variation, however. For example, the ovary of the mare is a very large, kidney-shaped organ. The ovary in dogs and cats is located in the dorsal abdomen. It will be found just caudal to the kidneys (see Figure 12.1).

The head of the uterus is connected to the body wall by the suspensory ligament. In dogs, this is a thick connection that requires some force to sever; in cats, the ligament is thin and can easily be broken with the finger.

The entire reproductive tract is suspended from the body wall by a thin, semitransparent membrane called the broad ligament. Although continuous throughout its length, the part suspending the ovary is known as the mesovarium.

The estrous (reproductive) cycle is dominated by hormonal control and will be elucidated later. On dissection, some small protrusions may be noted on the surface of the ovary. These are called follicles and contain the ova. They change in size throughout the estrous cycle and regress completely at some points.

In horses and cows, the follicles are easily rectally palpated during examination of the pelvis as part of a routine physical exam. This has great economic significance. For example, the presence and size of follicles in cows can indicate their stage of pregnancy. As one might imagine, the early stages of pregnancy in cows can be difficult to observe on gross examination of the animal. Particularly in dairy cattle, the discovery of pregnancy

Anatomy and Physiology for Veterinary Technicians and Nurses: A Clinical Approach, First Edition. Robin Sturtz and Lori Asprea.
© 2012 John Wiley & Sons, Inc. Published 2012 by John Wiley & Sons, Inc.

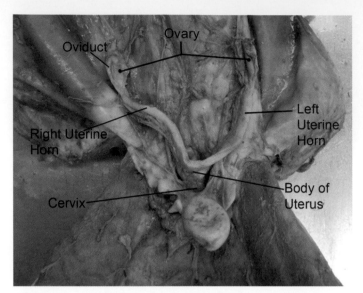

Figure 12.1   The female reproductive system. The animal's head is toward the top. The white pouch that appears to be caudal to the cervix is actually the urinary bladder, which has been reflected back from its normal position ventral to the reproductive tract.

Box 12.1   Boys and girls

Dog: male = dog, female = bitch

Cat: male = tom, female = queen

Horse: male = stallion, female = mare (neutered male: gelding)

Donkey: male = jack, female = jenny

Bovine: male = bull, female = cow (neutered male: steer; female who has not had a calf = heifer)

Sheep: male = ram, female = ewe (neutered male: wether)

Pig: male = boar, female = sow (neutered male: barrow; female who has not given birth to a piglet: gilt)

Goat: male = billy, female = doe (neutered male: wether)

Ferret: male = hob, female = jill (neutered male: gib; spayed female: sprite)

Rabbit (same terminology as for deer): male = buck, female = doe

and its relation to lactation is crucial to the commercial value of the animal.

Caudal to the ovaries are the oviducts. The ovum is funneled toward the ovary from the cranial end of the oviduct by the infundibulum, a hollow tunnel. It has a fringed end. These fringes are called fimbriae. In dogs, there is actually a small amount of space between the infundibulum and the oviduct. As a result of this, some ova can escape into the abdominal space.

The section of the broad ligament that suspends the oviduct is called the mesosalpinx. Note that the oviduct is relatively short compared to the next section, called the horn of the uterus. In most domestic animals, fertilization actually occurs within the oviduct, which is quite different from the process occurring in primates.

The oviduct on each side leads into a larger tunnel that proceeds caudally and medially. This section of the system is called the uterine horn. Dogs and cats, unlike primates, have a bicornate uterus. The section of the broad ligament suspending the uterine horns is the mesometrium, which continues to become the outer lining of the body of the uterus.

The fetal puppy or kitten actually develops within the horns of the uterus. After fertilization, the embryo comes to rest in the horns. As might be imagined, this tissue is highly distensible. While the horns of the uterus are relatively straight in dogs and cats, they loop extensively in sows.

The uterine horns meet at a common chamber called the body of the uterus. In dogs and cats, this area is very short. It is actually situated in a relatively more caudal position in cats than in dogs. This necessitates a different incision for ovariohysterectomy in each species.

The body of the uterus has an outer layer of connective tissue, with muscle tissue deep to it. The inner layer of the uterus is called the endometrium. It is a thick, layered, highly vascularized tissue. In cows, the embryo attaches to the endometrium via a structure called a caruncle.

The ovaries and uterus have strong vascularization and neural input, as well as a great deal of lymphatic drainage. The ovarian artery comes directly off the aorta and follows a torturous path.

The body of the uterus narrows as it travels caudally. A sphincter muscle called the cervix controls access to the uterus. The cervix stays closed except during some parts of the estrous cycle and during parturition. It has mucus-producing glands that assist in sealing the opening. The narrow area around and caudal to the cervix is known as the fornix.

The area from the cervix to the urethral orifice is known as the vagina. It is relatively thin and distensible, and courses through the retroperitoneal area. It has a smooth outer lining, with muscle and mucous glands within. It runs dorsal to the urinary bladder and urethra, and ventral to the rectum. There is a large venous plexus extending ventrally from the body of the uterus along much of the vagina, necessitating caution during abdominal surgery. Note that the possum actually has two vaginas, designed to accept the "double" penis of the male.

The urethra opens into the vagina at an area called the vestibule of the vagina. This resides caudal to the ischial arch and slopes toward the vulva, where the vagina/urethra exits the body. The vulva ends in two soft-tissue flaps called the labia, from the root word for lips. At the exit from the body is a structure called the clitoris. It has two parts and is the homologue of the penis (Box 12.2).

The male

The testicles (or testes) are the analogues of the ovaries (see Figure 12.2). They are smooth, solid, and ellipsoid in shape, and have approximately the same size in individuals of the same breed. Embryologically, the testes form in the cranial abdomen and descend to their location within the scrotum before birth.

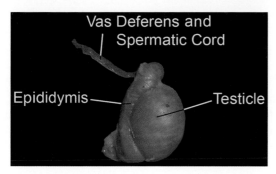

Figure 12.2   The distal portion of the male reproductive system.

Box 12.2   Babies

Dog: puppy
Cat: kitten
Horse: foal
Cow: calf
Sheep: lamb
Pig: piglet
Goat: kid
Rabbit: bunny, kit
Deer: fawn
Llama: cria

When the testicle fails to descend at the proper time, it may remain in an ectopic (abnormal) position. This condition is known as cryptorchidism. The problem is usually hereditary, so it is important that cryptorchid animals are not used as breeders. Unilateral cryptorchidism is most common, although bilateral abnormality is seen on occasion. The problem is solved surgically. Most often, the testicle travels as far as the area of the inguinal canal, close to the scrotum. It can, however, remain in the cranial abdomen. Therefore, removing it requires some searching to identify its location.

In some animals, the testicles remain within the abdominal cavity to achieve the proper temperature for the production of sperm. Pachyderms (elephants, hyrax) are an example of this type of system. In species such as most domestic animals, sperm must be produced at a lower temperature, so the testicles are located outside of the abdominal cavity. In some animals, for example, the bat, the testes descend at breeding season and then are retracted. Rabbits can retract their testicles at any time, which can make neutering a challenge.

In dogs and cats, the testicles reside within a sack called the scrotum. The scrotum has a median groove distinguishing one side from another. This division can result in asymmetrical sections. The skin is relatively thin and has many sweat and sebaceous glands. The testicles sit directly on the ventral scrotum. The scrotum can be alopecic, as in ruminants, sparsely haired, as in dogs, or heavily haired, as in cats. The muscle within the scrotum is the cremaster. The testes are suspended within the

scrotum at the end of the spermatic cord. The spermatic cord is a connective tissue tube that includes a large number of blood vessels within.

Another species difference has to do with the relative size and position of the testicles. In the bull, the long axis of the testicle is vertical, and the size of the testicle and scrotum relative to the size of the rest of the body is quite large. In contrast, the long axis of the canine testicle is horizontal, and its relative size is smaller. The testicles of the cat actually slant slightly toward the anus.

While the spermatic cord runs along one side of the testicle, the other side has a duct known as the epididymus. The external part of it is coiled. The testicles are covered by a connective tissue capsule. The epididymus and spermatic cord for each testicle run through a shared connective tissue covering.

The epididymus runs along the dorsal surface of the testicle in dogs, following a rather convoluted course. It is firmly attached to the testicle at the head and tail of the epididymis. The deferent duct emerges at the distal end of the epididymus and proceeds dorsally over the urinary bladder, through the prostate gland, and enters the urethra. The deferent duct is supported while within the abdomen by a peritoneal fold called the mesoductus. It is over the dorsal surface of the urinary bladder that the duct from each side joins to form one passage. The deferent duct carries sperm away from the testicle.

The spermatic cord contains the testicular artery and vein. There are a series of small veins that form a net-shaped structure called the pampiniform plexus. This condenses to a single vein that drains into the caudal vena cava. The testicular artery, like the ovarian artery, branches directly off the abdominal aorta. It too follows a contorted path to allow greater surface area.

Many mammals have what are known as accessory reproductive glands, which play an important physiological role. The prostate gland is present in dogs and cats. The bulbourethral gland is present in dogs but is vestigial in cats. The vesicular gland, which can be found where the deferent duct enters the urethra, is not present in dogs or cats. Of all of these, the one most likely to be seen on dissection is the prostate, which surrounds the urethra shortly after the urethra exits the urinary bladder. As in humans, enlargement of the prostate can either be benign or malignant. Prostate cancer in animals is much rarer than in humans but does occur.

The pelvic urethra (the part within the abdomen) is joined by the deferent and prostatic ducts and courses toward the outside of the body. It is highly vascular. It has a substantial layer of the urethralis muscle. The urethra runs ventrally to the rectum and can be palpated on rectal exam. In bovine practice, an instrument called an electroejaculator is inserted in the rectum to cause contraction of the urethra and to stimulate the discharge of semen; evaluation of sperm is critical in reproductive studies.

As the urethra exits the body via the penis, it is surrounded by an even more complex environment of vascular and erectile tissue. It courses all the way to the distal opening of the penis.

The penis is suspended from an area ventral to the trunk in most species, in the area of the caudal abdomen. A notable exception is the cat. The feline has the only rearward facing penis among mammals. It travels a relatively short distance once it emerges from the body.

The prepuce is the external protective layer of tissue around the penis. It is actually a fold of abdominal skin. It contains the free end of the penis. Within the penis are numerous vascular and lymphatic vessels, as well as erectile tissue.

Species differentiations are notable. In dogs, there is a small bone within the exterior penis, called the os penis. It is generally visible on radiography. In pigs and in some small ruminants, the penis has a prominent sigmoid flexure (S-shaped curve). Some species have a small protrusion of soft tissue at the distal end of the penis called the urethral process. The dorsal penis in the bull has an apical ligament holding it to the prepuce. If this ligament is too short, the penis deviates to one side on erection, making copulation unsuccessful.

Clinical case resolution: Canine orchiectomy

The cryptorchid dog represents a surgical challenge, to be sure. From the study of the growth history of the testicle, it can be determined that the testicle most likely has come to rest in the inguinal area as that is most often where its progress has been arrested. Therefore, a short incision would be made in that area and the search would begin. However, if not readily found, it may be necessary to extend the incision substantially toward the cranial abdomen. This can result in a surgery that is more time-consuming and extensive than a hysterectomy.

Review questions

1 What is the general term for a female cat?
2 What is the cranial-most part of the female reproductive tract?
3 What is the space between the ovary and the oviduct called (through which the ovum travels)?
4 The fetus develops in the _____ during pregnancy.
5 Do male dogs and cats have a prostate gland?
6 True or false: The male reproductive tract runs dorsal to the rectum in dogs.
7 What is a sigmoid flexure?

SECTION 2
PHYSIOLOGY

Chapter 13 The Cell

Clinical case: Blood glucose and brain function

There is a direct correlation between blood glucose levels and brain function. Hypoglycemic animals will often present neurological signs, such as seizures, as a result. What is the reason that glucose rather than another molecule has such an effect?

Introduction

While it is possible to consider matter at a subatomic level, and it can be argued that, in its own way, even this level of analysis relates to the function of all living (and other) structures, it is not really germane to our discussion. Therefore, to investigate the basis of physiology, it is best to begin at the level of the cell.

The cell is recognized as a microscopic entity having a border, a nucleus, and an internal power mechanism. This is not true of pathogens, for example; while they are microscopic, and many have a border, they may not have a membrane-bound nucleus (bacteria), or they may obtain the energy to exist by living inside another cell (viruses).

The cells that make up plants have a cell wall, which is to say that their border is less permeable and has materials not found in the borders of most mammalian cells. The matter of walls

becomes particularly important in considering bacteria; whether their borders are walled or not plays a role in how easy it is for antibiotics to penetrate them and disrupt their activities. This is one of the reasons that certain antibiotics are more effective against a given bacterium than others.

Mammalian cell boundaries

The borders of mammalian cells are circumscribed by a membrane, a structure more permeable (and more fragile) than a cell wall. The membrane is mainly composed of phospholipids. This has significant implications. Disease states that cause a phosphorus imbalance can disrupt the cell membranes themselves and lead to cell death. Drugs that are lipid soluble will penetrate the cells more easily than those that are not.

In fact, the metabolism of the entire body is dependent on the ability of materials such as gases (particularly oxygen) and nutrients to enter or exit the cell membrane. This occurs by way of a variety of transportation mechanisms. Materials can move in or out passively (move without requiring energy) or be escorted in or out (active transport).

One important concept when discussing transport into and out of a cell is that of osmosis. At its simplest, osmosis refers to the tendency of water and other molecules to be attracted to areas where the solution is concentrated. In a mammalian cell, the membrane is semipermeable. It does not let all molecules

Anatomy and Physiology for Veterinary Technicians and Nurses: A Clinical Approach, First Edition. Robin Sturtz and Lori Asprea.
© 2012 John Wiley & Sons, Inc. Published 2012 by John Wiley & Sons, Inc.

move in and out freely; if it did, it would soon be empty. If there is more material inside the cell than outside, water will be drawn in. On the other hand, if there is a great deal of material in the fluid around the cell, water will be drawn out. There is no energy required to make this occur. Osmosis is a type of passive transport, then, in that it does not need energy to work.

The production of energy

Living tissue, including bones, organs, and connective materials like skin, is composed of cells. Within each cell is a collection of structures that perform operations such as replicating genetic material and maintaining electrolyte balance. The cell requires energy in order to carry out these activities.

The mammalian cell performs both catabolism and anabolism. Catabolism involves breaking materials such as nutrients down into other materials that can be used by the cell. Anabolism occurs when the cell takes materials and combines them to make a new molecule. An example of the latter would be the cell using amino acids to build a protein.

The breakdown of glucose is accomplished by oxidation. In breaking down the glucose molecule, oxygen and carbon dioxide are produced. The complex series of chemical interactions that accompany this activity results in the production of adenosine triphosphate (ATP). The breaking of ATP by removing one phosphorus liberates a large amount of energy. This series of steps occurs in the cytosol (the liquid portion of the cell in which structures like the nucleus and mitochondria are embedded) and in the mitochondria themselves. Since oxygen is used, the process is called aerobic metabolism.

The reaction was first described by a scientist named Krebs, so the set of reactions is known as the Krebs cycle. The crucial element is that oxygen is required and that nutrients are converted into energy. The end result of the process is the incidental production of water and carbon dioxide, which are excreted.

Along with the conversion of nutrients into energy by chemical means, there are also changes in electrical charge. Ion exchange is a part of the process of producing energy. Electrons are replaced and removed at a regular rate, in such a manner that overall charge of the cell is not changed. The homeostasis (maintenance of a steady state to allow normal function) of any cell, or for that matter any body system, is what makes for normal function. In other words, the healthy state of the individual depends on maintaining a balance in many things, including energy production and ion exchange. When discussing the balance of charged molecules that involves oxygen, such as occurs in the production of ATP, the homeostatic balance is referred to as oxidation–reduction.

At its most basic, oxidation refers to the addition of oxygen, and reduction refers to its removal. The addition and removal are accomplished by way of chemical reactions using other molecules in the cell. When the reactions are carried out properly, the animal is said to be in redox balance (reduction/oxidation).

A consequence of oxygen deprivation is a disruption of normal energy production and, ultimately, cell death. One way we attempt to address this problem is to provide oxygen directly to the animal as a gas, to supplement his/her own respiratory system. Note that if oxygen is replaced too quickly or at too high a level, it can actually result in a flurry of activity that leaves an extra electron in the cell. This unbalanced negative charge can damage the cell significantly. If the blood supply to a previously poorly supplied area is restored too rapidly, or an animal in respiratory distress receives too much oxygen too quickly, more harm may be done than good. This is called reperfusion injury. It is important to be aware of this when working in an emergency or critical care area.

It is important that the animal have another way to make energy at times when oxygen levels are decreased. This decrease can be temporary (high levels of exercise, significant changes in altitude) or long term (as in disease states and/or injury). Energy production can occur without oxygen, in a process called anaerobic metabolism.

Aerobic catabolism uses materials such as glucose and its derivatives to make energy. The brain cannot use any other pathway to make energy than aerobic metabolism. It is for this reason that hypoglycemic puppies and kittens often show neurological symptoms; the brain cannot function without the oxygen and glucose it needs to make energy. Aerobic catabolism produces a large amount of energy.

However, there is a way to make low levels of energy, at a relatively fast rate, in some cells of the body. The anaerobic route of energy production also uses glucose; in fact, it can only use the sugars provided in food (as opposed to sugars produced as by-products of other metabolic activity). Muscle cells in particular are capable of anaerobic metabolism.

The drawback to anaerobic energy production is that a by-product called lactic acid is produced. Lactic acid is capable of damaging local tissue. During anaerobic metabolism, it can be converted to a less damaging molecule. However, if there is an overwhelming amount, it will be difficult or impossible to extract energy and to allow the process to continue. Muscle cramping can occur due to lactic acid buildup.

Muscle cells also use an anaerobic pathway that produces creatine phosphate. Creatine phosphate can be used to make ATP in the absence of oxygen. In addition, muscle tissue can store oxygen in the form of myoglobin.

Aerobic metabolism can continue uninterrupted if oxygen is available and the animal is eating. Anaerobic metabolism only occurs under specific circumstances. In either case, the organism is able to sustain energy production.

Clinical case resolution: Blood glucose and brain function

It is clear that glucose is a powerful source of energy for the survival of body cells. The brain itself cannot undergo anaerobic metabolism at all. If a low level of glucose in the blood persists, one of the most dangerous consequences is that neurological functioning will be adversely affected.

Review questions

1 What is the mammalian cell membrane mainly composed of?

2 Does diffusion into the cell require energy?

3 How does ATP relate to energy production in the cell?

4 True or false: The use of glucose for energy in a cell can only be accomplished if oxygen is present.

5 Can the brain use anything other than glucose for cell activity?

6 What does "redox" mean in relation to cell metabolism?

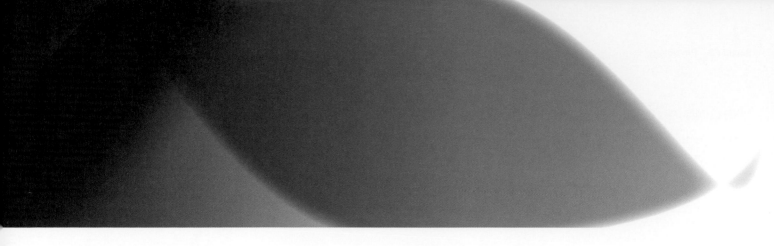

Chapter **14** Functions of the Common Integument

Clinical case: German shepherd with hair loss

A German Shepherd is brought into the clinic with areas of hair loss around the muzzle in the area of the nose and lips. The area is nonpruritic (not itchy) and does not have any discharge. On the list of diseases to consider is a rare autoimmune disease.

Introduction

The connective tissues that form the integument vary widely in appearance. We will consider some of the structures that accompany parts of the integument and their role in the life of the animal.

The phrase "connective tissue" is an umbrella term. It can refer to small areas of supportive material or to an entire class of structures. What they have in common is the presence of fibrous and/or ground substance. Ground substance refers to the scaffolding that contains specialized cells. For example, blood can be considered a connective tissue because it has a liquid base in which the active structures are carried and protected.

Connective tissue includes things like adipose (fat) tissue, mucous membrane, lymphoid tissue, cartilage, bone—and skin.

Skin

The skin has multiple functions. Among them are protection, thermoregulation, and maintenance of hydration. The protective aspects of skin become clear when there is a disease state or injury involving the skin. Gaps in the skin allow bacteria and fungi to enter, as well as environmental dangers such as parasites. The skin is an organ in that it has a series of functions in common throughout its structure. It is, in fact, the largest organ of the mammalian body. (The largest internal organ is the liver.)

There is a legend regarding the symbol of the veterinary profession, the Aesculapian. Unlike the caduceus of human medicine, the Aesculapian consists of a stick with a single wormlike creature ascending it. Supposedly, this represents a parasite commonly known as the guinea worm (named for the area in Africa where it was common). This parasite enters the human body when a person drinks contaminated water. It can travel within

Anatomy and Physiology for Veterinary Technicians and Nurses: A Clinical Approach, First Edition. Robin Sturtz and Lori Asprea.

the body for months as it matures. It is common for a given worm to exceed three feet in length. Eventually, a section of worm will emerge from the skin through a painful blister. Pulling at the worm would break it into small pieces, which potentially could get into, and then obstruct, the circulatory system. As a result, the common treatment was to wrap the end of the worm extending from the person's foot around a stick. The stick would be rolled slightly every day, so that the worm could be eased out of the body intact.

Thermoregulation

Mammals are able to maintain a constant internal temperature, regardless of outside temperature. This type of animal is referred to as a homeotherm. The opposite would be a poikilotherm, an animal whose body temperature varies depending on his environment. The temperature range in which the mammal's internal organs work is called "core temperature." As the name implies, the center of the body (heart and brain) must remain in this ideal temperature range. When temperature is measured, it must be remembered that the further away from the core of the body the temperature is assessed, the lower the temperature will be. Rectal temperature is closer to core temperature than is oral temperature, which is closer than axillary temperature (taken by simply placing the thermometer between the brachium and the axilla, occasionally done with very sick animals where an oral or rectal thermometer cannot be used). The rectal temperature level is easy to measure and is reasonably close to core temperature, so it is used most commonly in clinical practice. However, where great precision in measuring body temperature is needed, such as during surgery, a thermometer can be temporarily placed within the body.

An important structure of the skin that participates in thermoregulation is the sweat glands. Sweat glands form a fluid similar to saline that is discharged through a duct into the hair follicle, where it continues to the surface. The sweat approaches the surface of the epidermis and begins to evaporate. As it does, it cools the local area of skin. The discharge of sweat into the follicle is mediated by the autonomic nervous system (the series of neural commands that are delivered without conscious thought, but by automatic response to stimuli). There are also some sweat glands in hairless areas; these too are mediated by the autonomic nerves.

Water vapor is lost on exhalation. Panting is thus a useful activity to cause water evaporation. Cats generally do not pant to shed heat but use the other methods described to maintain body temperature. Evaporation is the main path to water loss as a method of temperature control. In fact, when the ambient temperature rises to approach body temperature, evaporation is the most effective natural method of heat control.

Another aspect of thermoregulation and the skin has to do with the concept of convection. When there is a significant difference between the air temperature and the temperature of the skin, with air temperature being cooler, air will flow away from the skin and lower its temperature. It is for this reason that puppies and kittens need to be kept in a warm area when new-borns. Their internal mechanisms for temperature control, mediated by the brain, are not mature at birth. The body thus is not able to avoid losing heat in a colder environment by convection, and temperature control must be maintained by other means (such as a nest or the mother).

Along the same lines, animals can also "insulate" each other. Close proximity allows the skin to share heat with others. Puppies and kittens, or animals in a cold environment, will huddle together in an attempt to maintain a normal working body temperature.

The skin contains sensory receptors for local temperature. These convey information to the hypothalamus, which has temperature-sensitive neurons. Information is then communicated, mostly by way of the autonomic nervous system, to engage in activities (sweating, shivering) to help maintain core temperature.

The haircoat also plays a role in thermoregulation by way of trapping cool or warm air close to the skin. The arrector pili muscles help raise the hairs, which enlarges the area in which air may be used as an insulating blanket. Once again, the arrector pili are mediated by the autonomic nervous system.

The subcutaneous layer of the skin is mainly composed of adipose (fat) tissue. Adipose tissue is an efficient insulator. Animals that live in cold climates, not surprisingly, have a thick layer of subcutaneous fat.

Another aspect of the thermoregulatory function of skin has to do with the concept of conduction. Skin in contact with, for example, a cold table or cold ground will lose heat. This is of particular importance if the patient is on a surgical table and under anesthesia. Most anesthetics slow the response of the central nervous system, including the activities relating to thermoregulation. With the ability of the body to regulate its internal temperature impaired, further loss by way of cooling of the skin is undesirable. As a result, most clinicians will place a warming device on the table or use a table with a built-in warming device. It is still necessary to assist with temperature control postsurgically until body temperature returns to normal.

Hydration

The adipose tissue of the body, particularly that of the subcutaneous layer, has an important function. It can hold a large supply of water. In the event that the animal is not drinking enough, or is urinating too much, the animal may be in the position of losing too much fluid content. The water content of the subcutaneous fat can then be called upon. An animal that is clinically dehydrated may lose even this backup supply. When this happens, the skin loses turgor (the normal full, firm condition of the tissue). In addition, the mucous membranes, particularly those of the oral cavity, may become pale and dry.

In clinical practice, we pinch the skin of the scruff and see if the skin bounces back into position. If it stays in a tent shape, it has lost the firmness that the water content affords. This is a quick way to assess dehydration. Loss of water content in the tissues supporting the globe can cause it to appear sunken into the orbit. This only occurs when dehydration is severe.

Clinical considerations

Other clinical indicators are provided by the skin and mucous membranes. The red blood cells contain a substance called hemoglobin. Hemoglobin is converted to bilirubin within macrophages of the spleen and liver. In addition, there is a large store of bilirubin in the liver that normally is discharged by the gallbladder as a constituent of bile.

In cases of destruction of red blood cells within the body, or in some hepatic diseases, free-floating bilirubin will build up in the bloodstream. These excess levels of bilirubin impart a yellow color to the skin, usually most apparent on the inner surface of the pinna, the sclera (white connective tissue visible on the surface of the eyes), and the mucous membranes of the mouth. Noting this color in any or all of these areas is an indication of either hemolytic disease (destruction of blood cells) or severe hepatic dysfunction. The condition is referred to as icterus.

As discussed in Chapter 8, the hemoglobin in the red blood cell carries oxygen to all parts of the body. As oxygen is released from the hemoglobin, it actually takes on a slightly blue tinge. This is particularly evident in the mucous membranes, which have a vasculature very close to the surface. Cyanosis is a condition denoted by a blue color in the mucous membrane or lips. Generally, by the time the condition is evident, there has already been a severe decline in blood oxygen content.

At times of hypothermia, or in injury severe enough to cause shock, the autonomic nervous system will cause constriction of the distal and superficial blood vessels in order to keep heat and oxygen close to the vital organs like the lungs and heart. Consequently, mucous membranes and the skin will become very pale. Pale mucous membranes are also associated with anemia.

sebum. Sebum contains sweat and oily secretions. Sebaceous glands provide a lubricating function and offer some waterproofing. The characteristic odor of a wet dog can be related to the production of sebum.

The circumoral glands are located along the lips, particularly toward the caudal part of the mouth. They are well-known in cats. Cats rubbing the side of their face against a person or an object are using the circumoral gland secretions to mark territory.

Carpal glands are sebaceous glands present in the carpal area of the cat. The location is marked by a tuft of tactile hairs.

Dogs and cats have tail glands, which are sebaceous glands located on the dorsal surface of the tail. As their activity is much greater during the breeding season, they are thought to play a role in advertising reproductive status.

Circumanal sebaceous glands are present in certain carnivores, and omnivores such as dogs. It is most likely the secretions of these glands that draw dogs toward introducing themselves by sniffing under the tail.

Sheep produce a substance from their sebaceous glands that is processed for human use. This material is waterproof as well as lubricating, and is occasionally used in cosmetics. It is known as lanolin. Musk deer produce a sebaceous product also called musk. This is used in perfumes for the human market.

The anal glands secrete a sebaceous material that lubricates and contains strong odors (see Figure 14.1). These odors serve as scent markers and are likely a functional analogue of the skunk's glands. In fact, when under severe stress, dogs and cats can actually expel the secretion toward the surrounding area. As noted before, the anal glands can become obstructed, leading to the phenomenon known as scooting. The animal is rubbing her hindquarters along the ground in response to the discomfort of the blocked gland. Anal glands can be "expressed" or emptied

Glands

The sweat glands are divided into two types: apocrine and eccrine. In both cases, a rather thin fluid is discharged, having a large supply of sodium. In fact, there is a minor contribution to electrolyte balance made by the sweat glands in this regard.

The apocrine glands discharge a fluid with a high protein level directly into the hair follicle. They are scattered throughout the body. As is true for eccrine sweat glands, there are species differences in how the glands are distributed.

The eccrine glands are those associated with hairless (or relatively hairless) areas of the skin. Their excretion is much more watery and plays less of a role in thermoregulation. There are many more apocrine glands than eccrine glands.

One other note, on a somewhat less scientific plane, concerns the degradation of sweat. Sweat in and of itself does not have a strong odor. What does happen is that the normal bacterial population of the superficial epidermis starts to degrade the sweat and then use some of its constituents. This is what produces a strong, rather musty odor.

The other glands related to the integument are the sebaceous glands. The sebaceous glands produce a waxy material called

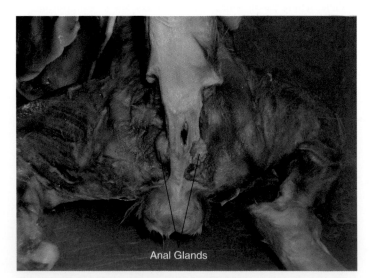

Anal Glands

Figure 14.1   In the living animal, the anal glands appear as a pinhole-sized opening on either side of the anus. This animal was an intact male, indicated by the size of the scrotum (just above the words "anal glands" on the picture).

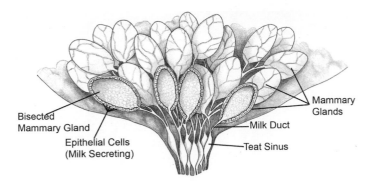

Figure 14.2   A cluster of mammary glands. Once the milk has entered the teat sinus, it can exit the nipple.

of their contents in the clinic. This provides instant relief for the animal. It does cause a strong, unpleasant odor, as anyone who has done the procedure will attest.

In addition, sebaceous glands assist the animal in scent marking by the production of pheromones. Pheromones are scents perceptible only to members of the same species (conspecifics). Pheromones are attractive odors and often have a calming effect. In addition, pheromones play a role in signaling reproductive status.

The mammary gland

The mammary gland is actually a type of specialized sweat gland. There are usually 8 mammary glands in two rows in cats and 10 in dogs. The gland has a complex series of ducts surrounded by fibrous connective tissue (see Figure 14.2). Eventually, the liquid content, to which fats and proteins have been added, exits via the teat.

The number and location of teats vary widely. Primates have two, located on the ventral thorax. Equines have two, located in the inguinal (groin) area. Dogs have a variable number, but usually have four to five on each side of the ventral thorax and abdomen. Note that several canals lead from a number of glands to converge on one teat; that is, when the neonate is nursing, each teat is discharging the product of a cluster of glands. It should also be noted that while males have mammary glands, they do not lactate. The teats of a male mark the location of their glands, but the glands do not enlarge unless there is some illness. While most male mammals have teats, rats do not.

In the first 24 hours or so after a puppy or kitten is born, the mother's milk is referred to as colostrum. This is because it contains a collection of maternal antibodies, protecting the infant from at least some infectious diseases until the young animal is able to make its own antibodies. This process is known as conferral of passive immunity.

The flow of milk is governed by a number of factors. The nuzzling of a nursing newborn will set off a series of cues that alert the pituitary gland to release oxytocin. Oxytocin stimulates "milk letdown." This refers to the muscle contraction and ductile constriction that are associated with the passage of milk from

the teat. Nursing (or milking by hand) also leads to the release of prolactin, which helps maintain lactation. Growth hormone is required for milk production. It was felt that giving dairy cows growth hormone would increase their output of milk; the administration of this hormone is controversial in that there is concern as to whether the growth hormone might affect humans drinking milk from these cattle.

Note that the production of milk actually begins before parturition (birth). The milk is stored in the alveoli (microscopic areas connected by ducts, resembling the alveoli of the lungs). This first milk is the substance known as colostrum, which contains maternal antibodies that support the infant's immune response. Lactation, which is the action of making the milk available to the newborn, occurs immediately before or during parturition. In fact, the presence of progesterone and estrogen, which are pregnancy-related hormones, actually inhibit lactation. When these factors no longer are present, lactation can proceed.

While milk letdown is usually stimulated by suckling, there are other ways to accomplish the discharge of milk from the mammary gland. The most familiar one is using manual pressure on the nipple, otherwise known as milking the animal. While commercial milking usually involves goats and cattle, any mammal can be milked (with a reasonable amount of cooperation from the animal).

Hair

The haircoat in most mammals sheds in whole or in part. The difference among them has to do with time frame. In primates, shedding occurs throughout the year. In most domestic animals, shedding occurs at particular times of the year.

As a single hair begins to grow, the follicle will project it above the surface of the epidermis. At some point, as the season of shedding begins, the hair follicles will begin to atrophy. As they atrophy, the hair maintains its position. As a new follicle begins to grow again, the hair is pushed out of position and loses its connection to the follicle. In other words, it falls out. This does not happen all over the body at once. Similarly, birds molt in patches throughout the body and do not lose all of their feathers at the same time.

In dogs and cats, the hairs that form the top layer of the coat are called guard hairs. They usually grow in long layers, with the occasional whorl or border. This factor facilitates the protective layer of the coat. For example, in the rain, the water will tend to "sheet" off the animal and thus provide some protection for it. Note that some species are bred to have different patterns of hair. While this may arguably improve their appearance, it actually does deprive them of some protection from the elements. So-called hairless breeds suffer not only from temperature extremes but also from damage related to extended exposure to ultraviolet rays or dampness.

As an aside, hair does not serve only to keep an animal warm. Haircoats can trap cool air as well, and in some breeds, leaving the haircoat on is more advantageous than shaving it off in hot weather.

The undercoat, made of so-called wool hairs, is generally more contoured. Wool hairs are shorter than the guard hairs. As noted in Chapter 2, these are the hairs that shed when an animal is combed. Loose wool hairs can wrap around each other, particularly in long-haired dogs and cats, and cause painful knots known as "mats," short for matted hair.

The tactile hairs extend above the guard hairs and below the wool hair follicles. Some tactile hairs can be traced down to the level of the muscle. These follicles are surrounded by a venous sinus (cuplike opening) lined with mechanical receptors that communicate with local nerve fibers. Thus, anything that touches the tactile hair will be perceived as movement and will thus command attention.

Whiskers are the classic example of tactile hairs, but there are others. For example, a cluster of tactile hairs marks the location of a sebaceous gland in the area of the caudal carpus in the cat. Whiskers are rarely shed and are quite hardy. The facial whiskers are known as vibrissae, most likely in recognition of their sensitivity to vibration. In fact, the vibrissae should never be trimmed except in cases of medical necessity, as this is quite bothersome to the patient.

The pads

The pads of the paw are very thick, cornified (dead) epithelium. There is a thick layer of collagen and elastic fibers, combined with some adipose tissue (fat) that underlies this. The pads perform a protective layer for the animals, regardless of the kind of surface upon which they move.

The stance of the animal determines which pads are in contact with the ground. The three stances in mammals are plantigrade, digitigrade, and unguligrade.

In plantigrade stance, the entire palmar and plantar surfaces are in contact with the ground; that is, the paw, caudal metatarsal/metacarpal area, carpus and tarsus are all in direct contact with the surface while the animal is moving around. The classic examples of this are rabbits and kangaroos. Thus, there are digital pads, metacarpal/metatarsal pads, and carpal or tarsal areas that meet the ground when the animal walks.

Dogs and cats have what is called digitigrade stance. This means that the digital pads make contact with the ground. There is a single metacarpal pad on each forelimb, and a similar metatarsal pad, and these too contact the ground. The carpal pad serves no purpose. There is no corresponding tarsal pad.

It is untrue that dogs and cats do not sweat. The pad contains, in its subdermal layer, a few sweat glands. The mark of a nervous cat in the examination room is the appearance of damp footprints as the animal walks across the table. These glands are more related to sympathetic nerve stimulation and territorial marking than they are to thermoregulation.

In ungulates, only the digital pad is in contact with the ground. In ruminants, the digital pad is called a bulb. In horses, it is called the frog. Given that the horse stands on one digit only, it is not surprising that the digital pad is quite stiff and complex in structure.

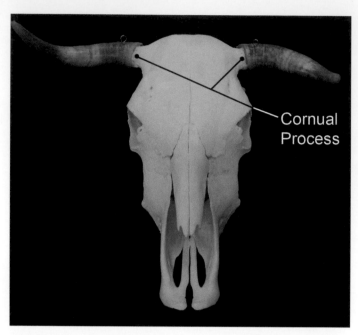

Figure 14.3   Horn grows out from the cornual process. In bovines, the interior of the process actually communicates with the interior of the skull.

Antlers and horns

Although we are primarily concerned with dogs and cats here, we would like to briefly discuss antlers and horns. Both are composed of epidermis and have a dermal layer (see Figure 14.3).

Antlers are outgrowths of the skull. As they protrude, they are covered with skin. The skin dies as it is stretched continually and is referred to as velvet due to its smooth appearance as it hangs from the prongs of the antler. The exposure of the bone to the elements causes it to die, and the antler falls off. The shedding of antlers, like the shedding of hair, is usually seasonal, responding to changes in temperature and length of day. Seasonal changes will incite the antler to grow again.

Horn grows from the cornual process of the skull. Horns grow continuously from the time they appear, which is shortly after birth. At first, there are small button-like growths called horn buds, which are relatively easy to remove if there is some reason to dehorn the animal. Horns grow in length and width as the animal ages. In cattle, the interior of the horn actually is continuous with the frontal sinus, a hollow area rostral to the dorsal braincase. When animals are dehorned, it is particularly important to avoid any debris falling into the cavity and to use aseptic technique in order to lessen the risk of sinus infection.

Clinical case resolution: German shepherd with hair loss

The German Shepherd described above had lesions at the mucocutaneous junction. Literally, this is the border between the mucous membrane and the skin, such as that found at the border of the nares. An autoimmune disease called systemic lupus erythematosus is often first diagnosed when the described lesion is identified. Happily, it is a rare disease in animals.

Review questions

1 What is convection (in the context used here)?
2 Define poikilotherm.
3 What are the muscles that control the hair follicles?
4 What is the proper name for the whiskers?
5 The mammary glands fall into what category of glands?
6 Define pheromone.
7 What is the difference between horns and antlers?
8 Name a species that has digitigrade stance.

Chapter 15 Osteology

Clinical case: Bone marrow biopsy in a German shepherd

A German Shepherd comes in for a yearly examination. The client reports that the pet is "slowing down lately" and has a decreased appetite. Testing of the blood reveals an abnormal count of white blood cells. When repeated testing shows the same problem, and no clear cause is evident, the doctor decides to do a bone marrow biopsy and chooses the iliac crest for this.

Introduction

The major bone groups of the mammalian body are the long bones, the short bones, the irregular bones, and the flat bones. The bony structure of the animal, the skeleton, does not serve only for support and protection of the interior organs. The skeleton also plays an important role in movement through its interaction with joints and serves as the site of blood cell production and mineral storage.

The growth of bones

The lengthening of long bones (such as the femur) while the young animal grows occurs at either end of the bone rather than in the middle. If the middle of the diaphysis (shaft) of a long bone is marked, that mark will not move, even as the animal grows "taller." The growth area is in the metaphysis, caudal to the articular surface of the bone. In the young animal, a plate of cartilage is present at its border with the epiphysis. This epiphyseal plate is gradually converted into mature bone by the action of cells called osteoblasts.

It is important to note that the epiphyseal plate does not appear when bone is radiographed as cartilage is mostly transparent to X-rays. An X-ray picture (radiograph) of the long bone of a young animal will appear to have a separation between the ends of the bone and the diaphysis. This is sometimes mistaken for a fracture.

Bone cells do eventually get broken down by cells called osteoclasts. They need to be replaced, and so while the bone does not get longer after a certain age, there continues to be growth within the bone itself. The activity within the metaphysis continues until adulthood. The material within the metaphysis is called

Anatomy and Physiology for Veterinary Technicians and Nurses: A Clinical Approach, First Edition. Robin Sturtz and Lori Asprea.
© 2012 John Wiley & Sons, Inc. Published 2012 by John Wiley & Sons, Inc.

cancellous bone. It consists of softer materials like bone marrow. It has a spongy appearance. Flat and irregular bones actually have cancellous bone as well, although their growth patterns are different.

The way bone grows is of particular concern when there is a fracture. As the bone rebuilds, the osteoblasts (cells that become mature bone cells) start to repair the damage by creating woven (disorganized, immature) bone first. The collection of this material is called a callus. The callus consists mostly of fibrocartilage, a relatively soft material. This will take a while to become mature bone. For this reason, severe fractures require immobilization of the area. Excessive movement will interrupt the building of the new bone.

Mature bone is called compact bone. This is very durable and usually forms the outside wall of the bone. Compact bone is composed of a series of microscopic structures called osteons, which are a round series of layers with a central canal through which blood vessels flow. The osteons form a strong platform for the bony structure. Note that compact bone contains things like collagen and other proteins, and minerals like calcium and phosphorus. Cancellous bone does not have osteons but instead has a ladder-like series of intersecting cells. Cancellous bone is always covered by a thin layer of compact bone (see Figure 15.1).

The storage of calcium and phosphorus is important to the animal for use in energy production, and bone may be called upon to supply them if the usual stores of calcium and phosphorus are not sufficient. Calcium and phosphorus imbalance can be caused by diet, endocrine, or renal problems.

In essence, the parathyroid gland is the part of the endocrine system that contributes to balance of the electrolytes calcium and phosphorus. If the animal is hypocalcemic (low levels of calcium in the blood), parathyroid hormone (PTH) will be released by the parathyroid glands. PTH mobilizes calcium from the bones by inducing it to enter the bloodstream. Another hormone, calcitonin, blocks the discharge of calcium from the skeletal structure.

Note that vitamin D derivatives play a role in the activities of PTH. Vitamin D is important for other reasons as well. It is a key player in helping the gastrointestinal (GI) tract absorb calcium from the nutrients traveling through the tract. Some of that calcium goes to help build and maintain the bone.

Some animals undergo a negative calcium balance, meaning that they are losing more calcium than they are taking in. This can become a serious problem in milking cows. If they lose too much calcium in the milk they are excreting, they can develop hypocalcemia (low levels of calcium in the blood). The body is unable to mobilize enough calcium from its reserves to fill in the gaps, and the animal suffers severe weakness. The condition is fatal if not addressed promptly.

Bone marrow

While there are small areas of marrow in other bones, the long bones contain the bulk of the bone marrow in mammals. Bone marrow is present in the medullary cavity of the bone. Bone

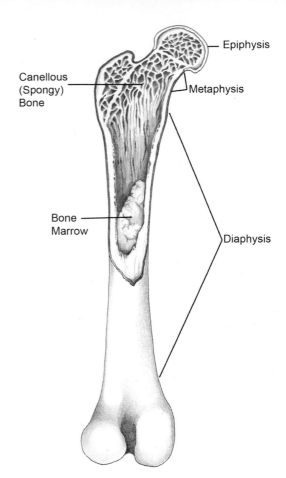

Figure 15.1 (1) Epiphysis, (2) metaphysis, (3) cortical bone, (4) endosteum, and (5) bone marrow.

marrow produces most of the blood cells the body uses. As the animal gets older, some of the marrow cells are replaced by fat cells. The mature animal is still capable of producing new blood cells but at a reduced rate. The areas around the head of the humerus and the head of the femur continue to actively produce blood cells. It is for this reason that in cases of decreased white or red blood cell levels in the blood, we will usually check the bone marrow's ability to produce them by sampling from the humeral or femoral head.

Flat bones have marrow that continues to be active throughout life. Another place that bone marrow is sampled is from the ilium, for this reason. This is usually done in dogs only. In cats, the ilium is relatively thin and less sturdy, and it can fracture during the procedure.

The difference between cartilage and bone is that cartilage, while it is a connective tissue, has no ossified material in it; that is, it does not have a hard matrix of osteons. It also does not have blood vessels or nerves running into it as bone does. Cartilage receives its nourishment not from the blood directly but from diffusion (passive transport) of nutrients from local vessels through the interstitium into the cartilage.

Cartilage

There are three main types of cartilage: hyaline, fibrocartilage, and elastic cartilage. Hyaline cartilage is composed mostly of collagen, a protein common in the structure of connective tissues like bone and skin. It is the type of cartilage that lines the surface of bones where they meet a joint. Hyaline cartilage in the normal animal should have a smooth appearance and should be pink in color (slightly yellow in older animals). Excessive use and/or injury can cause the cartilage to wear down or tear, resulting eventually in inflammation and abnormal gait.

Fibrocartilage is a thick form of cartilage with strands of protein called fibrin running through it. An example of fibrocartilage is the material that makes up the articular labrum (lip around a joint fossa). The labrum helps prevent friction as the femur moves. Fibrocartilage has tremendous tensile strength. Subsequent to injury, fibrocartilage may replace hyaline cartilage.

Elastic cartilage bends freely. The pinna of the ear is an example of elastic cartilage. It provides shape but allows the tissue to be mobile as needed. Another example of elastic cartilage is the epiglottis, which covers the vocal cords and moves aside as needed to let sound and air escape.

Ligaments, tendons, and joints

Ligaments and tendons are made of connective tissue. Tendons are much thicker and, as a result, are supportive of a large range of movement. Tendons are both elastic and strong, which suits them to the work of connecting bones across joints, or muscles to bones or other muscles. Tendons do not have their own blood supply. As a result, injuries to a tendon do not heal well as they are poorly supplied with materials to rebuild.

Tendons and cartilage play a role in the movement of the skeleton. The joints are areas where one bone meets another. Note that not all joints are mobile. The sutures of the skull, while not completely solid in the fetus, do not move in the adult animal. They are made of fiber and are called immobile joints because they represent an area where different bones meet, but no change in position between the bones occurs.

Most joints are involved in movement to some extent. The synovial joints have the greatest range of motion. They are located where a great deal of movement is required, or where there is a need to change the angle or direction of motion quickly. Thus, the coxofemoral (hip) joint and the stifle joint are synovial joints. In order to speed up body movement through space, the body needs to "push off" from a given spot to build up momentum. Synovial joints allow that kind of movement.

Round or crescent-shaped structures made of fibrocartilage are present in many synovial joints. Each is called a meniscus, and they cushion the bones as they move back and forth. There are several in the stifle and one at the temporomandibular joint on each side.

Many of the joints of the limbs work on a principle similar to that of a lever. The range of motion of the limb depends on its balance point and on how far that point is from the joint, just like the range of motion of a seesaw depends on how far the person is seated from the center of the apparatus. This principle is applied to orthopedic studies, including investigation into methods of physical therapy for animals such as dogs and horses.

Avians

Chapter 3 considered the concept of the pneumatized bones of the avian. The spaces within the bones are arranged such that the ossified (bony) parts run at angles to each other as well as in parallel fashion. This provides a strong scaffold, particularly for the powerful muscles involved in flight. It also serves to lessen the animal's weight so that the bird can fly more successfully. (Nonflighted birds also have pneumatized bones, although the bones may not be as completely pneumatized, and thus may be heavier, than those of flighted birds.)

Other adaptations to flight include the presence of the air sacs (see Chapter 23), which allow efficient breathing while keeping the body weight low. The tibiotarsus is essentially one long piece, which provides greater stability when standing, given that the dorsal part of the animal weighs relatively little.

As mentioned earlier, feathers are a type of epidermis. The general category of feathers include contour and down feathers. Contour feathers are those on the exterior of the bird. Specialized contour feathers called primaries and secondaries are most involved in the aerodynamics of flight, helping to control direction and height while airborne. When referring to "clipping the wings" of a bird, the procedure is not that of removing the wings, but of trimming the primary contour feathers such that the bird cannot fly very high or very far. This is a protective procedure for some captive birds. The down feathers are mostly related to insulation.

Clinical case resolution: Bone marrow biopsy in a German shepherd

As noted, blood cells are mostly made in the bone marrow. Sampling the bone marrow will allow us to determine if the count is abnormal there as well. The iliac crest provides a good place to take a bone marrow sample if the animal is big enough in that it is easy to access. In this particular case, the dog turned out to have an abnormal number of cells in the bone marrow as well, indicating that the production of the cells (rather than loss of cells through, e.g., internal bleeding) is the problem. Unfortunately, this animal turned out to have cancer (lymphoma).

Review questions

1 True or false: We can only sample bone marrow from long bones and not flat or irregular bones.
2 If a year-old animal suffered a wound from buckshot and a pellet remained in the center of the femur after the injury,

would it still be in the same position (if it was not surgically removed) in 5 years? Why?

3 What is the epiphyseal plate composed of in the newborn puppy or kitten?

4 The outmost, fibrous layer of a long bone is called the _____.

5 What is compact bone?

6 What does an osteoclast do?

7 Do ligaments and tendons have blood vessels in them?

8 What type of cartilaginous material covers the articular surfaces of most bones connected by joints?

9 True or false: The temporomandibular joint does have a meniscus, but only one for each joint.

Chapter **16** Muscle Physiology

Clinical case: Body condition score

One way of measuring the relative condition of an animal is to look at his body condition score. Graded on a scale of 1–5 (or 1–9), it gives the clinician an idea as to how healthy the animal is. One of the first things to happen when an animal is inappetent is a decreased body condition score. The relationship will become clear at the end of this chapter.

Introduction

Musculature is certainly a mechanism for locomotion. However, among their many other functions, muscles are involved in respiration, the cardiovascular system, and the digestive system. They play a role in the sensory systems (particularly vision and hearing). In short, complete failure of muscle function is not compatible with life.

Locomotion

The gross appearance of the skeletal muscles is an important part of a physical exam. Severe weight loss sometimes even affects the appearance of the muscles themselves; they will atrophy if they cannot sustain their normal energy level.

Recall that the structure of skeletal muscles, which provide the primary force for voluntary movement, includes bundles of fibers called fasciculi. Each muscle fiber is made up contractile structures called myofibrils. Skeletal muscle cells have multiple nuclei.

Terminology regarding muscle cells is different. Structures may have different names, although they often serve the same function as the analogous parts in other cells. For example, the fluid part of the cell within its membrane is referred to as sarcoplasm, just as the interior of a somatic cell is called cytoplasm. In place of the endoplasmic reticulum of other cells, the phrase is sarcoplasmic reticulum. In both cases, the structure is responsible for channeling material around the interior of the cell. The cell membrane is called a sarcolemma. It is no surprise, then, that a type of muscle tumor is referred to as a sarcoma.

The muscle fiber is composed of a series of light and dark bands that are parallel to each other. It is this alternate series of bands lying on top of one another that give rise to the striated appearance of the muscle. The darker bands are referred to as thick filaments and the lighter ones as thin filaments.

Both the thick and thin filaments are composed of protein. The thick filament is composed of a protein called myosin. The

Anatomy and Physiology for Veterinary Technicians and Nurses: A Clinical Approach, First Edition. Robin Sturtz and Lori Asprea.
© 2012 John Wiley & Sons, Inc. Published 2012 by John Wiley & Sons, Inc.

thin filament is composed of actin. Smaller proteins called troponin and tropomyosin are also present in the thin filament. These proteins play a role in the contraction of the muscle fiber.

The generation of adenosine triphosphate (ATP) is particularly important in the process of muscle contraction. The ATP comes from a series of steps involving the oxidation of glucose and the processing of phosphates. A lack of glucose-containing nutrients will lead to abnormal muscle function. The lack of glucose (or abnormal glucose processing) can lead to twitching of muscles (muscle fasciculations). There is a particular risk of this in puppies and kittens, which do not have a mature glucose processing system. Note, however, that muscle can make energy from other sources as well if need be.

A store of ATP is present in muscle cells, but it needs to be replenished. The major ways that muscles do this are by using the cell's store of creatine phosphate, breaking down glucose, and cellular oxidation of nutrients. Note that important features are glucose and oxygen. This explains the need for animal athletes to have a high-energy diet and why high levels of activity cause a need for increased oxygen.

The issue of creatine phosphate is also clinically significant. An animal that is losing a significant amount of weight will have some damage or atrophy to the larger muscles, usually those of the trunk at first. High blood levels of an enzyme called creatine kinase are associated with muscle damage and/or significant weight loss. This can be useful, particularly when a client is not sure how long the animal has been losing weight. If a client is new to the clinic, there may be no record of the animal's prior weight. The combination of an increase in the creatine kinase level in the blood and evidence of muscle atrophy is reflected in the body condition score (BCS).

A dog or a cat in good body condition will have a slight waist, ribs that are not easily visible but are palpated easily, and no large areas of fat deposits (unless part of the animal's breed characteristics). An animal in that condition would be given a score of 3 out of 5 (written 3/5), or 5 out of 9. The higher the number, the more overweight the animal is. The lower the number, the more underweight the animal is. The condition called cachexia refers to a person or an animal with severe, globalized muscle atrophy and prominent bone structure. The condition is usually associated with cancer or severe chronic illness. We would judge an animal like this as having a 1/5 BCS. Keeping track of these scores each time the animal gets a physical exam will help the examiner recall what the animal looked like before.

The generation of a muscle contraction

In Chapter 18, a full discussion of the neurological side of the stimulation of muscles is covered. The point at which the nerve meets the muscle is called the neuromuscular junction. The nerve fibers that provoke skeletal muscle activity are called motor neurons. They contain the neurotransmitter acetylcholine (Ach). The Ach opens the channels that allow sodium and potassium to enter and leave the cell, respectively. (This exchange allows for the changes in cell voltage that make the transmission of the nerve impulse possible.)

When the nerve impulse reaches the sarcolemma, a number of things happen. Primarily, the actin of the thin filaments actually bends toward the myosin of the thick filaments. As they are drawn toward each other, ATP acts to push them apart again. This, in turn, allows the next set of filaments to go into action. The filaments slide back and forth against each other as a function of all of this activity. This movement is what leads to the contraction of the muscle fiber.

In addition to sodium and potassium, a major electrolyte involved in the function of the muscle fiber is calcium. There are small conduits called T-tubules that are present near the cell membrane (sarcolemma) and end near the sarcoplasmic reticulum. When a nerve impulse is received at the muscle fiber, the sarcoplasmic reticulum will release calcium, which is stored within the reticulum (from the Latin word for network). The liberated calcium is then channeled into the T-tubule, where it binds with troponin. The stimulation of calcium-bound troponin causes a conformational (shape) change in the tropomysin. This exposes a site on the actin where the myosin can bind. ATP provides the energy needed to release the myosin from this site; the myosin then travels further along the chain, setting off a wave of muscle contraction, as described above. If the muscle is stretched, the filaments will slide so as to lengthen the muscle fiber. The reverse is true for the contraction of the muscle. The calcium is escorted back into the sarcoplasmic reticulum when the neurological stimulus stops.

There actually is always a low level of muscle tone, even in a stationary animal; that is, the majority of skeletal muscles are held in a "ready" state by being slightly contracted or extended. This is what allows animals to maintain a particular body shape and to respond to any need for sudden movement.

Note that action potentials come along rapidly once they are started. The speed with which the exchange and movement of electrolytes, and the actin–myosin reaction, take place is enough to allow repeated movement of the muscle fiber. Until an enzyme (in this case, acetylcholinesterase) breaks down the neurotransmitter completely, the neuron will continue to fire, and the muscle cells will respond. Therefore, two mechanisms are used to stop muscle contraction: depleting stores of ATP and interfering with the interface of the neurotransmitter with its receptors in the sarcolemma.

The number of muscle cells stimulated by a single neuron (based on the number of dendrites it has) is called a motor unit. In some cases, a single neuron may stimulate a very small number of muscle fibers. In others, a neuron may cause a large section of a muscle cells to stretch or contract. The fewer muscle fibers a single neuron connects to, the more specific the muscle response; that is, if a single neuron controls a single fiber, very fine control over the movement of that muscle is possible. It is a little like using a bowling ball: If you push the ball just a little bit at a time, you can very precisely target a specific pin. If you throw the ball with full force from one end of the lane to the other, you will hit a number of pins but may not topple the one you want. The more motor units associated with a given muscle, the less precise the muscle movement. On the other hand, the muscle will be capable of much stronger force because it has so much innervation.

The basis of speed

Muscle fibers can be described as either "slow twitch" or "fast twitch." Slow-twitch fibers are also known as "red" muscle, as a result of their high level of myoglobin (an oxygen-bearing compound that lends a red color to the muscle). Fast-twitch fibers are correspondingly lower in myoglobin and are referred to as "white" muscle. The reason the terms slow and fast are used is that the neurons that innervate these muscles are either of small diameter or large diameter. Small-diameter neurons have a slower transmission of the action potential, and larger-diameter neurons a faster transmission.

This has a bearing on our clinical practice in that it helps us understand why some animals can maintain a high level of activity for a short period of time, or a lower level of activity for a longer time. Note that if a sustained level of high energy is required, anaerobic metabolism may be necessary. The buildup of lactic acid that accompanies this is responsible for the sensation of a muscle cramp.

The slow-twitch muscles are best for endurance; they produce a sustained level of energy, albeit at a slower pace. This kind of muscle serves a bird in flight quite well. Avian flight can be over very long distances without fatigue because the muscles are not being asked to come up with a sustained rapid pace.

A strong release of high-energy movement that lasts only a short time utilizes the fast-twitch fibers. Watching a lion hunt down prey will reveal this pattern. The lion can put on a tremendous explosion of energy, running quickly and covering a great deal of ground. However, the lion cannot keep that up for too long. If the prey can stay away from the predator long enough, the predator will have to stop to rest, and the prey can move further away.

Smooth muscle

The lack of striations in the outward appearance of smooth muscle reflects the fact that these muscle fibers are shaped like a spindle rather than straight lines. They do have thick and thin filaments, as do striated muscle fibers, and the mechanism of actin–myosin interaction is similar. The series of steps that are involved in this cycle go at a much slower rate. This lower rate consumes energy at a much lower level.

As a result, smooth muscle can maintain a constant or slowly changing state of relaxation or contraction. This serves an important function: smooth muscles are associated with actions like change in the diameter of blood vessels and contraction of muscles associated with the gastrointestinal (GI) tract. These are

functions that go on, constantly or intermittently, throughout each day. Unlike skeletal muscles, which are only called upon during voluntary movement, smooth muscles require continued activity. In fact, many smooth muscles are called into action while the animal is asleep or relatively inactive. They maintain a constant tone, or low-level activity, on a much greater level than skeletal muscle does. The gastrocnemius muscle is only active at times the animal is moving the pelvic limb. The muscles controlling the saphenous vein's walls go into and out of function regardless of the animal's state and without the animal's conscious awareness.

Smooth muscles do not rely strictly on motor neuron circuits. The autonomic nervous system has a primary role in contraction or relaxation of smooth muscles, using different neurotransmitters to stimulate motor movement. These neurotransmitters include norepinephrine and nitric oxide. Ongoing research into the function of nitric oxide as a messenger is the basis of research into current and potential pharmacological treatment of disease.

Hormones have a direct influence on the function of smooth muscles. For example, the reproductive system responds to the pituitary hormone oxytocin. Oxytocin causes contraction of the smooth muscles associated with the uterus, as well as the mammary glands.

Other chemical messengers play a role. The substance histamine, an inflammatory chemical carried by basophils (a type of white blood cell) and by mast cells (another inflammatory cell), will be released in the presence of allergens. Another type of white blood cell called an eosinophil is able to cause the release of histamine. Histamine causes contraction of the smooth muscles of the respiratory tract.

Cardiac muscle is different in that it has a striated appearance throughout most of its tissue. However, there are areas of smooth muscle. The smooth muscle components with their sustained capacity for work are important in a muscle that absolutely must keep functioning for the animal to live. On the other hand, the ability to provide very forceful contraction, with bursts of energy as needed in emergencies, requires the efficient use of large amounts of energy associated with striated muscle.

The striated fibers of the heart muscle are branched. The branches are separated by small gaps which can be crossed by the nerve impulse. The eventual outcome of this arrangement is the ability of the fibers to undergo synchronous contraction, meaning that all fibers contract at the same time.

Intercalated disks are structures known as tight junctions, which allow the heart to undergo strong contraction without tearing the muscle apart. The branches of striated muscle cells serve to increase the surface area of the fiber while spreading out the force of the contraction.

While the heart generates its own action potential, it is also governed to some extent by the autonomic nervous system. The effect is to ramp up or dampen the ongoing strength of contraction as needed (e.g., to step up the rate and force of the heartbeat if a predator on the hunt occurs). This will be discussed further in Chapter 20 ("Cardiovascular Physiology").

Clinical case resolution: Body condition score

Recall that the epaxial muscles are the superficial muscles of the dorsum. They are rapidly affected by a lack of nutrients. Thus, when an animal is not eating well, these are among the first muscles that lose mass (atrophy). When an animal's vertebrae are felt readily, or even seen, on physical examination, we give a low body condition score. This reflects our concern regarding the animal's health.

Review questions

1 True or false: Actin and myosin are types of proteins.
2 The main neurotransmitter associated with the neuromuscular junction in skeletal muscle is _____.
3 While waiting to be used, calcium is stored within a muscle fiber in the _____.
4 Smooth muscle is governed mostly by the _____ nervous system, and its main neurotransmitter is _____.
5 Is it more important for skeletal muscle or smooth muscle to maintain a continuous level of activity?
6 Would the administration of epinephrine have more of an effect on the skeletal muscle or on the smooth muscle?

Chapter **17** Sensory Physiology

Clinical case: Brachycephalic dog

A brachycephalic dog comes into the clinic with her people. They are quite upset and report that the dog seems to have trouble seeing. Upon examining the eye, the clinician finds that the intraocular pressure is very high.

Introduction

The sensory receptors are the cells that capture the stimuli from the outside world or elsewhere within the body and communicate them to nerve fibers. They are clustered within sense organs, specialized structures containing neural tissue that can be concentrated in a small area, or spread along in a series of clusters, such as in the tactile system.

Receptors

Some receptors accept stimuli that come from a distance. For example, the visual system is designed to capture information

from not only its immediate area but also from feet or even miles away. Contact sensory systems such as taste and touch are those that require proximity in order to function.

The sensory systems include the visual, auditory (hearing), vestibular (balance), olfactory (smell), tactile (touch), and gustatory (taste) receptors. These systems take information in from outside the body. Each system includes the receptor cells and their surrounding tissue. While they vary greatly in structure, each gathers information and projects it toward the central nervous system, where the information is processed and acted upon.

There are also internal receptors, which give the central nervous system information about the workings of body systems and metabolism. These include baroreceptors and chemoreceptors, which will be discussed later.

The nature of sensory receptors governs how the information is processed. A given system may interpret any stimulation as if it belonged to the class of stimuli to which it is responsive. Applying pressure to the eye will often cause an impression of a visual image, even though there is no specific material to "see."

Receptors are classified according to the nature of the input to which they respond. They include photoreceptors, auditory

Anatomy and Physiology for Veterinary Technicians and Nurses: A Clinical Approach, First Edition. Robin Sturtz and Lori Asprea.
© 2012 John Wiley & Sons, Inc. Published 2012 by John Wiley & Sons, Inc.

receptors, mechanical receptors, chemical receptors, and thermoreceptors. In order, they respond to light, sound, physical contact, chemicals, and temperature. In fact, sensory organs actually have the ability to filter out information that they do not respond to. They also have a threshold; that is, stimuli have to reach a certain strength in order for the receptor to respond.

The thresholds for various stimuli vary by species. The auditory system of dogs and cats responds to a different range of sounds than that of primates. In turn, other species use completely different systems in order to carry out the same functions. Bats have minimal capacity to receive visual images. However, their refined auditory system serves the function of informing the central nervous system of the size and location of objects.

In addition, most sensory systems are adaptive; that is, they have some method of coping with too much (or too little) information. The mammalian eye can perform certain functions to limit the amount of light impinging on this sense organ so that it is not overwhelmed (e.g., constricting the pupil of the eye). Movement of the pinna can help amplify local sounds to make them easier to hear.

The sensory information that impinges on the receptor organ generates a response in local nerve fibers. This is known as transduction. An action potential (neural signal) will be triggered when enough input from the fibers is received. This is called integration. The series of action potentials reflect the intensity of the input. If the input from the environment continues, the strength of the action potential will increase. If the input intensifies, the impulses usually will come more frequently.

If the stimulus continues past the ability of the receptor to keep up with it, or if the stimulus is less startling as it continues, the response of the neural system actually decreases. This is known as receptor adaptation. A cat may respond strongly to the sound of an air conditioner being turned on. However, as the sound continues, his auditory system adapts, and the response lessens.

The visual system

In the early stages of evolution, cells sensitive to light were present in various locations. In dogs and cats, those cells are now clustered in the eye, an organ that uses both neural and structural enhancements to accept visual input

Structures of the eye

In looking at the mammalian eye, we are struck by a number of complicated structures. From the outside, the most prominent feature is the eyelid, or palpebrum. The upper and lower lids meet at a "corner" called the lateral canthus on the lateral side of the globe (eyeball), and the medial canthus near the nose. There is actually a "third eyelid," properly called the nictitating membrane, folded under the ventral palpebrum in the area of the medial canthus. It is made of stiff, fibrous material and will sometimes protrude if the animal is unwell. It contains a gland

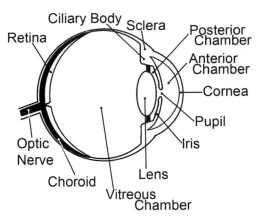

Figure 17.1   The parts of the eye. The anterior and posterior chambers are filled with aqueous humor, and the vitreous chamber with a much thicker fluid called vitreous humor.

that helps produce tears. There is a duct at the medial canthus that conducts tears into the nasal passage. Blockage of the tear duct is not uncommon and can be tested by placing a dye into the duct at the medial canthus and seeing if the dye runs out of the nose.

The outermost part of the eye is the cornea, a transparent membrane covering the globe (see Figure 17.1). Between the cornea and the iris is the anterior chamber, which is filled with a thin fluid called aqueous humor. The white part of the eye is called the sclera. It is made of dense fibrous connective tissue. The iris is the colored part of the eye. In an animal which is an albino (lacking in the cells that make pigment, or color, for the connective tissues such as skin), the iris is usually pale pink. The opening through which light travels is the pupil. Immediately caudal to the iris is the ciliary body. This structure produces the aqueous humor and assists in focusing the lens.

Between the iris and the lens of the eye is the posterior chamber, also filled with aqueous humor. The lens is held in place by a number of suspensory ligaments called zonules.

Behind the lens is the vitreous body, a thick gelatinous material that helps the globe retain its shape. The part of the globe caudal to the lens is called the vitreous chamber. The vitreous humor also serves to press against the retina and hold it in place. On dissection, the vitreous humor appears as a puddle of viscous gel within the globe. The aqueous humor, on the other hand, will retain its watery appearance and volume.

The retina is a many-layered stack of cells that processes light so that the brain can attach meaning to the images. The retina contains the cells that distinguish light and dark, and shades of color. Deep to the retina is the retinal pigmented epithelium, a layer of specialized cells. This, in turn, sits on the choroid, which is the vascular layer of the eye. The choroid contains the tapetum lucidum, which in the living animal appears blue or green when one looks into the globe with an ophthalmoscope. On dissection, the tapetum often appears dark blue or green. Primates and swine do not have a tapetum lucidum. The glow of an animal's eyes when light is directed toward them in a dark room, or outdoors at night, is the reflection of the tapetum.

Function of the eye

Muscle fibers in the iris are arranged both radially and circularly. This allows the pupil to allow in more or less light. This movement is controlled by the autonomic nervous system. During anesthesia, we can judge how much effect the drugs have had by looking at the dilation of the pupil. As the pupil comes down to a more normal size, we can infer how much the neurological system has recovered from the anesthetic agents.

There are also muscles caudal to the iris, in the ciliary body of the posterior chamber. These help alter the conformation of the lens of the eye, allowing the animal to change its ability to focus. This accommodation allows for readjustment for near and far vision.

The ciliary body has another important function. It participates in the production of aqueous humor. Under normal circumstances, the aqueous humor flows from the choroid through the pupil and into the anterior chamber. Aqueous humor is then drained out of the eye at the junction between the iris and the cornea. This location is called the iridocorneal angle. If the production of aqueous humor is abnormally high, or the flow of the aqueous humor is blocked, the condition known as glaucoma results. This condition is an unrelieved increase in intraocular pressure caused by the larger than normal amount of fluid in the eye.

The retina has a number of layers. The photoreceptor layers are those that contain the cells called rods and cones. The rods are dedicated to responding to levels of light. The cones are sensitive to things like color and detail. As an aside, it is not true that dogs and cats are insensitive to color. The range of colors they see is most likely different from that of primates.

The tapetum lucidum reflects light strongly within the eye, helping to enhance the strength of the visual signal. The combination of the size and reflective quality of the tapetum, and the degree to which the pupil can open, makes some animals much better at distinguishing visual images in low light. Nocturnal animals demonstrate these qualities to a great degree.

The information gathered by the retina is transmitted by way of nerve fibers to the optic disk, which is where the fibers are gathered to form the optic nerve (cranial nerve II). The optic nerve is unique in that its fibers are actually directed along its trunk in different directions. For example, some information from the medial portion of the retina of each eye follows the optic nerve as it crosses from right to left or left to right at the optic chiasm. However, information from the lateral part of each retina stays on the same side of the body as it travels along the optic nerve. This splitting of the fibers allows the visual cortex to make very precise calculations as to the position and strength of visual stimuli.

Another aspect of visual processing relates to the nature of the image. The visual image that the eye receives is inverted as it passes through the lens and the fluids of the eye. It passes through the optic nerve in this upside-down position and is not rotated to a "normal" position until it reaches the visual cortex of the brain.

There is a difference in the placement of the eye in predator and prey species. Most predators have eyes placed rostrally or at least close to the center of the muzzle. The fact that the eyes are relatively close together helps the animal focus and improves its depth perception. Prey animals tend to have eyes placed more laterally. This allows them to have a wider range of vision, including the ability to see more of the area to the side and even a little behind them. This is a clear advantage in sensing prey. However, it also means that the animal has much less depth perception and that it does not see well when it is approached directly from the front. Partly for this reason, it is best not to approach an animal like a horse directly from the front, so as not to startle it, unless one makes a noise or touches the animal or otherwise indicates one's presence.

Proprioception

Proprioception is the ability of the body to orient itself in space and to sense its direction of movement. Proprioception depends on the integration of information from a number of systems. Visual images and the relative expansion and contraction of muscle groups help the body determine its position and the direction in which parts of it are oriented. The component of the system that is related only to the sense of balance is actually a part of the inner ear called the vestibular apparatus. It senses information regarding balance and position in space. Figure 17.2 has information regarding the structure of the vestibular and auditory portions of the inner ear.

The semicircular canals and vestibule of the inner ear contain a viscous fluid called endolymph. Floating in the endolymph are small solid crystals called otoliths. As the body moves, the

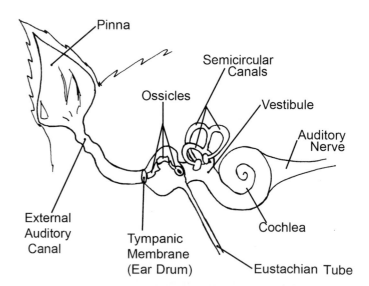

Figure 17.2   The area from the pinna to the tympanic membrane is the outer ear. From the tympanic membrane to the cochlea is the middle ear, housed in the tympanic bulla. This includes the Eustachian tube. The cochlea, semicircular canals, and vestibule form the inner ear; the latter two relate to proprioception.

otoliths move. They come to rest on cells that have small cilia on their luminal surface. The mechanical act of the cilia being bent by the otoliths coming to rest on them triggers a response in the local nerve fibers, which lie at the opposite end of the ciliated cell. The fibers conduct the impulse as they gather together to form the vestibular part of the vestibulocochlear nerve (cranial nerve VIII). The vestibular nerve meets the auditory part of the nerve, which exits from the cochlea, and they continue to the auditory cortex (located in the temporal lobe of the brain). Infection or tumors of the inner ear or cranial nerve VIII can result in impaired function of the balance mechanism. The most common symptom of this problem is head tilt, where the animal is unable to keep its head in an upright position. The other symptom sometimes seen is nystagmus, which is a rapid side-to-side or up-and-down movement of the globe. It can be seen on gross examination of the living animal, particularly if the examiner tilts the patient's head back. The presence of nystagmus reflects the close association of the visual system and the inner ear in maintaining balance.

The auditory system

The sense of hearing is facilitated by a number of anatomic, mechanical, and neurological features. It begins with the pinna in most mammals. In most dogs and cats, the pinna is not only relatively tall but is also somewhat mobile. In turning the pinna slightly from one side to another, sounds can be gathered in more directly. The pinna not only gathers the sound but also amplifies it, albeit very slightly. The length and width of the pinna relative to the size of the head is one factor in its amplifying capability. The "oversized" appearance of the pinnae of the bat contributes to the ability to sense and locate sound.

Sound is conducted from the pinna down the external auditory canal to the tympanic membrane. The strength of the auditory signal is reflected in the degree to which the tympanic membrane vibrates. The speed of the vibration of the sound waves (associated with whether the sound is low or high in pitch) is also transmitted in the movement of the tympanic membrane. The common name of the tympanic membrane is the eardrum, in deference to its similarity to the head of a drum.

The vibration of the tympanic membrane, in turn, sets off the vibration of the ossicles. This continues the transmission of the signal. The footplate (flat part) of the most medial ossicle (the stapes) sits in a membrane-covered opening called the oval window. This window is actually an opening into the cochlea, the part of the inner ear that has to do with hearing. The ossicles are housed within the tympanic bulla. Normally, the bulla does not contain any fluid. Infection in the nasal passages can enter the bulla by way of a tube connecting the nasal cavity with the bulla (middle ear). This tube is called the Eustachian tube. Medial to the bulla is the cochlea, which looks like a snail shell. It is the cochlea that is properly called the inner ear, not the bulla. Therefore, most bacterial or yeast infections of the ear (the most common type of ear pathogens) actually are in the external ear canal, with a few in the middle ear. An infection of the inner ear can only be called such when the infection is located within the cochlea or vestibular apparatus (balance mechanism).

As the stapes vibrates, it sends a pressure wave through the fluid within the cochlea. This fluid wave sets off movement that leads to stimulation of the receptor cells within the cochlea (which are also ciliated cells). As in the balance mechanism, the deflection of the cilia set off changes within the receptor cell that trigger a neural impulse. The action potential ends in the temporal lobes of the brain, where the information is processed.

The olfactory system

Particularly for animals whose hearing and/or vision is not very acute, the sense of smell needs to be very keen. The olfactory system houses some receptor cells that are specialized, responding to a particular odor, and some that are general, responding to a variety of smells. Many olfactory cells are ciliated.

There are special receptors for pheromones. The importance of these species-specific olfactory stimuli is reflected in the fact that they have their own receptors. Pheromones are particularly important in the reproductive cycle and in territoriality. A female in heat produces a particular pheromone to advertise her condition to others of her species. Males will often mark their territory with pheromones secreted by some sebaceous glands.

In felines, the vomeronasal organ presents an opportunity to enhance smells. The organ is a collection of soft tissue with receptor cells that is located near the nasal cavity. When air is drawn somewhat forcefully across this area, the olfactory bulb is stimulated. The reader may have observed a cat sniffing an object and then standing still with its mouth slightly open. What it is doing is drawing air across the vomeronasal organ to make the olfactory stimulus stronger.

Olfactory receptors are induced to produce an action potential when they are stimulated. These potentials are brought directly to the olfactory bulbs, which are the rostral-most part of the cerebrum.

The gustatory system

The tongue of most mammals is the primary sense organ for taste. Specialized cells in the tongue respond to tastes such as sweet and sour. Some species respond only to very few tastes in that their taste receptors only categorize materials into a couple of general categories.

It is difficult to specify what tastes appeal to a given individual animal. For example, it is felt that cats do not have a strong response to sweet tastes. However, some felines clearly prefer sweet-tasting foods. How they interpret the taste is, of course, difficult to assess; what tastes sweet to us may taste sour to them. Unfortunately, the main chemical constituent of automotive antifreeze is ethylene glycol. This chemical appears to have a sweet taste to dogs and cats, and dogs will readily consume it if it is available. Ethylene glycol is very damaging to the kidneys and can be fatal.

The tactile system

The distinguishing feature of the sense of touch is that it combines mechanical and neural signals to transmit information. Stretch receptors within the skin sense physical pressure, and thermoreceptors indicate changes in temperature. The ability to feel pain is referred to as nociception and is signaled by the inflammatory response. The latter refers to the fact that certain proteins and white blood cells are recruited when there is injury or infection. These materials also set off a cascade of neural responses that cause the central nervous system to interpret them as aversive.

Specialized receptors

Throughout our discussion of physiology is the theme of feedback loops and self-monitoring of biological systems. Two receptor cell clusters that are linked to cardiovascular and respiratory functions deserve mention here. They are the baroreceptors and chemoreceptors, cells that sense blood pressure and carbon dioxide, respectively. They will be discussed in greater depth as we go along. For now, it is important to note that sensory input occurs from within the body as well. The information obtained from these receptors is used by the nervous system to adjust the activities of the cardiovascular and respiratory systems.

Clinical case resolution: Brachycephalic dog

It is unfortunately the case that certain breeds, because of human manipulation of their gene pool, have a high incidence of certain diseases. The conformation of the head that certain breeds of animals have fits into this category. Brachycephalic (flat-faced) dogs have many problems related to the eye; the shape and position of it do not always fit well with the orbit and the rest of the skull. As a result, it is not uncommon to diagnose glaucoma in breeds such as the bulldog. Glaucoma is a condition under which the fluid pressure rises in the eye. This condition can be painful and can eventually cause blindness if not treated.

Review questions

1 What is the proper adjective for the sense of taste?
2 Define proprioceptive.
3 True or false: The semicircular canals are structures involved in both hearing and balance.
4 The ossicles are contained within the outer, middle, or inner ear?
5 What is the tapetum lucidum?
6 What is the name of the fibrous white part of the eye just deep to the cornea?
7 True or false: Some fibers of the optic nerve cross to the other side of the brain, and some stay on the same side.
8 What is the vomeronasal organ?

Chapter 18 Neurophysiology

Clinical case: A puppy dragging one limb

A puppy is brought into the clinic. He is awake, alert, and seems to be normally active. However, he is dragging his left thoracic limb. The only significant history is that the puppy had blood drawn by a breeder (who is not legally permitted to do this).

Introduction

To maintain homeostasis, the body must be able to "read" its status with regard to every organ and body system (including the brain itself). Neurological physiology involves the propagation of a signal along each nerve cell, bringing information to or taking information from cells or groups of cells throughout the body. Along with hormones, nerve impulses are mediators of metabolism. From the management of cardiac and respiratory functions to the governance of the olfactory sense to the ability to play catch, the nervous system is crucial.

Information from outside the body must be gathered, delivered to the central nervous system (CNS) (the spinal cord or the brain, or both), and then acted upon. For an illustration of the spinal cord, see Figure 18.1.

The neuron

The neuron, or nerve cell, is composed of a cell body, projections called dendrites, and a relatively long extension called an axon (see Figure 18.2; this illustration also appears earlier in this text). Neurons can deliver information directly to each other but more commonly communicate with cells outside the neurological system. An average mammalian vertebrate has 10 billion neurons. In large animals, a single axon can be 1 m long.

Note that the neuron itself needs energy in order to function. It depends strictly on glucose (e.g., as opposed to lipids) in order to generate energy. The use of glucose to produce energy requires the presence of oxygen. As has been discussed, the CNS cannot use anaerobic energy systems. This is why oxygen deprivation has such a catastrophic effect on the nervous system. It is also the reason that hypoglycemia (low blood glucose level) affects the nervous system.

Energy created by variations in electric charge propagates along the axon, like ripples in a pond, until it can be handed off to the next cell. The stimulation of this energy pulse is what

Anatomy and Physiology for Veterinary Technicians and Nurses: A Clinical Approach, First Edition. Robin Sturtz and Lori Asprea.
© 2012 John Wiley & Sons, Inc. Published 2012 by John Wiley & Sons, Inc.

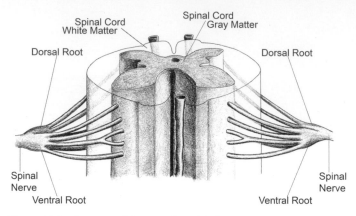

Figure 18.1   Sections of the spinal cord (schematic).

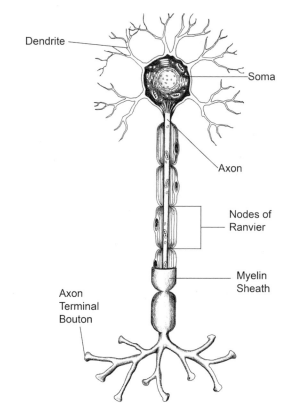

Figure 18.2   The neuron. Not all neurons have myelin. The nodes of Ranvier are locations where there is no insulation covering the nerve fiber itself.

provides the platform for launching the activity of the destination cell.

The soma is the body of the nerve cell, and the axon the long projection coming from it. The thicker the axon, the faster the nerve impulse can travel. Some axons have a sheath of fatty tissue called myelin, which insulates the axon.

Note that afferent signals are the ones that bring sensory information from the rest of the body (or from outside the body) to the CNS; efferent signals are those heading from the CNS to another destination. In the spinal cord, neurons conducting afferent signals have their soma in the dorsal root ganglion of the spinal nerves. Efferent fibers, some called motor neurons, usually have a soma in the CNS, with axons going out to the muscles, glands, or other organs. As will be noted below, the architecture of the autonomic nervous system is somewhat different.

When a nerve impulse, called an action potential, arrives at the soma, it can cause the production of another action potential, which travels along its axon to propagate the message. The distal surface of the axon is known as the axon terminal, or the terminal bouton. The axon terminal can direct its energy to another axon, a dendrite, or a cell in the organ or tissue being stimulated (known as the target tissue). For example, if the trigeminal nerve (cranial nerve V) is bringing a signal to the muscles of the jaw, those muscles would be the target of that nerve.

Transmission across the synapse can be chemical or electrical. In mammals, the vast majority of transmitters are chemical. In other words, the axon terminal releases a chemical across the presynaptic membrane when the nerve is stimulated. This chemical travels across the synapse, arrives at the postsynaptic membrane (i.e., the next cell in the chain), and stimulates an activity that varies depending on the nature of the target. These chemical messengers are called neurotransmitters.

The action potential

The action potential is the wave of electrical energy that is propagated along the axon and releases the neurotransmitter. It is particularly dependent on the electrolytes sodium and potassium. Disease states that disrupt the levels of these ions can seriously impact neurological function. In addition, potassium is the basis of some of our euthanasia drugs; excess of potassium will fatally interrupt nerve impulses and muscle function, causing the heart to stop.

The resting potential of a neuron is the electrical charge within the cell relative to the electrical charge in the tissue around it. The area around the cell is relatively more positively charged. The slightly negative charge within the cell is referred to as its "resting potential." In domestic mammals, that charge is −75 mV.

The extracellular area contains less potassium and more sodium than the intracellular area. Using the energy caused by the production of ATP within the cell, potassium can be pumped outside of the cell, bringing sodium in. The reverse can also occur. The process is called the Na-K-ATPase pump.

Depolarization occurs when this ion exchange makes the interior of the cell less negative. The use of the phrase "less negative" is deliberate; the charge may rise to −50 mV, for example, which is still negative, but less so than −75 mV. When it returns to its resting (usual) potential, the process is called repolarization.

A neuron at rest has a minute electrical charge. The charge changes when the neuron is stimulated by another neuron or by chemical interchange. When this happens, channels will open within the axon.

Sodium in the surrounding tissue takes advantage of this to rush into the neuron. As sodium is a positive ion, the amount of negative charge decreases. Once all the channels open, there will be a large surge of electrical energy, kicking off the response along the rest of the axon. However, with all the channels open, potassium (which is also a positively charged ion) goes out of the cell. Since there is usually less potassium surrounding the cell than in it, the potassium within the cell is drawn to an area where it has more room.

In short, the neuron uses glucose as a fuel to produce energy. That energy kicks off an exchange of sodium and potassium that changes the electrical charge of the cell.

As the neuron returns to its resting potential, it usually "overshoots" the mark. In other words, instead of returning to the resting level of $-75\,mV$, it will go to an even more negative level, say, $-95\,mV$. This overshoot is referred to as hyperpolarization. The amount of time it takes to get back to the resting level is known as the refractory period. During this time, the neuron cannot respond to another stimulus even if it receives one. Not all neurons, therefore, fire at the same time.

Nerve impulses vary in both the speed and the frequency at which they travel. In mammals, the flowing series of electrical changes can travel at $20–100\,m/s$, and there can be more than 100 impulses per second.

The nodes of Ranvier are areas along myelinated neurons where there is no myelin covering. As with a bare wire, the electrical charge can jump across those areas rather quickly. This forms an efficient way of propagating the action potential. Diseases that cause demyelination, or the destruction or lack of the myelin sheath, cause severe neurological abnormalities. Demyelinating disease in dogs is quite rare. In humans, perhaps the most familiar one is multiple sclerosis.

The generation of the excitatory potential (stimulating a neural response) will set off a cascade of ion exchange along the length of the axon until it reaches the end. Bear in mind that nerve impulses can be inhibitory as well; they can slow or interrupt a message or body function.

The distal-most part of the terminal bouton is called the synaptic terminal. The axon from which the signal comes is the presynaptic terminal, and the cell that receives it is designated as the postsynaptic terminal. In discussing the function of the autonomic nervous system later in this chapter, the question of presynaptic and postsynaptic fibers will assume particular significance.

As mentioned before, the axon of the neuron is a projection of the cell itself. Among other things, this means that its cytoplasm is the same material as that in the soma. In addition, it means that its membrane surrounds not just the terminal bouton but also the entire neuron.

Neurotransmitters are chemicals that transmit messages to the postsynaptic neuron, allowing it to undergo depolarization. The number and types of neurotransmitters vary tremendously; only some of them will be discussed here. The use of neurotransmitters, natural or synthetic, to control nerve impulses is an area of intense interest and research in searching for new medications. Drugs that can mediate these reactions can help control the metabolism to an impressive degree.

Once neurotransmitters, such as acetylcholine, cross the synapse, they impinge on the cell membrane of the postsynaptic neuron. These neurotransmitters stimulate small openings to emerge at various places along the membrane. These openings are called channels.

The specific cause of channel opening depends on the type of channel it is. Ionotropic receptors are those that open in response to voltage change. This reaction causes the channel to open and accept charged particles such as sodium. This allows the ion exchange that triggers the next action potential. The entire reaction is based on the voltage on either side of the membrane. Ionotropic channels form the basis of the action potential propagation along the axon.

Another type of receptor is known as a ligand-gated channel. These channels are paired with a large molecule (receptor) that functions as a dock or receiving area. The receptor has a particular size and shape. Thus, only a certain transmitter can link up with this channel, by way of the receptor. The binding of the neurotransmitter to the receptor forces open the channel and allows ion exchange. Unlike a voltage-gated channel, ligand-gated channels do not depend solely on voltage differential. If enough neurotransmitter comes along, it will bind to the ligand and gain entry into the cell. More neurotransmitters will cause more channels to open. These channels are found in large numbers at the postsynaptic axonal membrane.

Having crossed the synapse and caused the channels to open on the postsynaptic membrane, the neurotransmitter will either be destroyed or returned to the point of origin. If it were to stay in the synapse, the target cell would be constantly bombarded with energy and would not be able to "turn off." This can be turned to advantage in designing medications for use in neurological or neuromuscular disorders.

Central and peripheral functions

From a functional standpoint, the nervous system is divided into two parts. The CNS is composed of the brain and the spinal cord. The peripheral nervous system is, essentially, all the other nerve fibers (neurons). In general, peripheral nerves carry information toward and away from the CNS. There are, of course, blood vessels and supporting tissue affiliated with both sections of the nervous system.

Some transactions involve sending information to and from the spinal cord and not to the brain. In particular, responses called reflexes often are mediated by the spinal cord alone. The patellar (myotactic) reflex is commonly assessed to investigate suspected neurological damage affecting the pelvic limb. A sharp tap of the patellar tendon generates a nerve impulse that travels to the spinal cord. The spinal cord, in turn, sends a message to the limb, causing the stifle joint to flex. The brain is not involved in this activity. The brain can be functioning perfectly, but damage to the spinal cord may prevent the reflex from occurring. In fact, we use this information to help determine if signs of neurological disease are related to problems in the brain, or caudally.

The CNS has an integrative function; it takes input from various sources and systems and generates a response. For example, information from the auditory and visual nerves can be analyzed. If the result of the analysis is that a bear is coming after the dog, the brain can send the motor neurons into action, stimulating the dog to, say, run away.

The peripheral nervous system has sensory components, called afferent nerves, which bring information from elsewhere in the body to the CNS. The motor neurons, which bring instructions to various body systems, are known as efferent nerves.

Much of the animal's sensory input (sound, taste, visual images, odors, tactile sensations) travels to the brain stem and is then projected on to the hypothalamus. Through the control the hypothalamus can exert over the autonomic nervous system, it is able to direct the activities associated with thermoregulation, systemic blood pressure, stress responses, reproductive hormones, and the digestive system. Many of these functions involve the endocrine system, which is discussed in Chapter 22.

The hypothalamus has other functions as well. For example, it senses levels of electrolytes (sodium, potassium, calcium) and induces the pituitary and adrenal glands to help control these levels. It also helps monitor blood glucose. Using information from the eye, it helps control the circadian rhythms. The circadian rhythms are a type of internal clockwork that uses the 24-hour day as a base. Cycles like temperature regulation and the sleep/wake cycle depend in part on the function of this part of the brain.

The brain

The brain itself can be described in a number of ways. A common way of approaching the subject is to divide it into three parts. These are functional divisions, not physical ones.

The forebrain includes the cerebrum. It contains the thalamus and the hypothalamus. It also includes the hippocampus, a part of the brain devoted to learning and memory, and the limbic system, where emotions are processed.

The hindbrain includes the cerebellum. The cerebellum governs motor movement and the autonomic nervous system. Kittens exposed to the virus causing panleukopenia prior to birth (in other words, if the mother is infected) often develop cerebellar hypoplasia. This literally means that the cerebellum is undersized and abnormally shaped. These kittens walk abnormally and may have other neurological signs.

The midbrain refers to all of the sensory integration areas within the brain. These are the areas where sound, light, and tactile information are processed (see Figure 18.3).

The cranial nerves are those that emanate as a trunk (large collection of nerve fibers) from the brain and travel directly to the target of interest. See Appendix 2 for their names, numbers, and functions.

The autonomic nervous system

The peripheral nervous system itself is divided into two parts. One is the somatic system, which is involved with voluntary responses such as skeletal muscle movement. The other is the autonomic nervous system. In its resemblance to the word "auto-

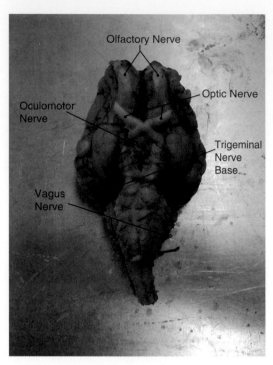

Figure 18.3 The vagus and trigeminal nerves exit the brain stem. The optic nerve comes from each side of the head and crosses at the optic chiasm. The rostral-most parts of the ventral brain are the olfactory bulbs.

matic," it may be apparent that the autonomic nervous system relates to activities of the body that do not require conscious thought. This covers functions of the smooth muscle, such as is present in the blood vessels, various glands, and the cardiovascular and respiratory systems.

The autonomic system is further divided into the sympathetic and parasympathetic systems. They have opposing functions under most conditions; one speeds things up while the other slows them down. See the accompanying box for more information.

Most efferent autonomic nerve fibers originate in the hypothalamus. As they travel along, they exit the CNS and head toward their destination. The part of the nerve that exits the CNS is called a preganglionic fiber.

Once the nerve fiber reaches the ganglion, it stimulates a soma. Axons go out from there to the target tissue or organ. These latter fibers are called postganglionic. The distance of the ganglion from the origin of the fiber is different for the sympathetic and the parasympathetic systems, but the concept of the structure is similar.

The sympathetic nervous system is often called the "flight or fight" system. When an animal is startled, stressed, or otherwise exposed to a strong stimulus, it will either run away or confront the source of the stimulation. The ability to do this requires a number of responses. There will be an increased heart rate to bring more circulating blood to the organs that are now in need of great amounts of energy. The bronchi expand to allow in more oxygen. The functioning of the urinary and intestinal systems is changed so that they are less active; wasting energy on urinating or digesting while trying to escape a predator is less than convenient.

The parasympathetic system is known by the phrase "sleep or eat." When the animal needs to rest, the parasympathetic nervous system brings the heart rate back to normal (or even slows it). When the animal is at rest, the digestive system is at the ready when food is available.

The sympathetic nervous system relies mostly on norepinephrine to carry messages from one nerve fiber to another. Nerve fibers that use norepinephrine as a neurotransmitter are referred to as adrenergic fibers. Fibers that release acetylcholine as a neurotransmitter are called cholinergic fibers. There are some in the sympathetic system, although the vast majority are in the parasympathetic system.

Receptor cells within the sympathetic nervous system fall into two basic categories: alpha receptors and beta receptors. In general, alpha receptors are present when excitation is called for. Stimulation of beta receptors will usually inhibit or decrease the function of the cell they are associated with. A drug that enhances the function of alpha receptors, then, would be useful in stimulating activity. Many of the drugs we use, particularly in the cardiovascular system, have to do with blocking or enhancing the function of these receptors.

The parasympathetic system, as mentioned a moment ago, uses acetylcholine to transmit information from one nerve fiber to another. Cholinergic fibers can bind to one of two types of receptors: nicotinic or muscarinic. The muscles have many nicotinic fibers. (People who smoke are well aware of the relationship between nicotine and involuntary muscle tremors.) Muscarinic receptors are present throughout the parasympathetic nervous system. They are present in large numbers in the heart and help to slow the heart rate down.

It is noteworthy that the gastrointestinal tract has its own intrinsic nervous system, referred to as the enteric nervous system. Both chemical and mechanical (stretching) activities in the stomach set off these nerves, which control the moving "wave" called peristalsis that brings the ingesta along through the intestines.

The urinary bladder has both sympathetic and parasympathetic innervation. When the sympathetic system is not actively engaged, the parasympathetic system will respond to expansion of the urinary bladder as it fills with urine and contract to expel the urine. Recall that there is skeletal muscle (voluntary) control of the exit of urine as well; this is what allows an animal to urinate only in certain places or under certain conditions, such as going out for a walk with a human.

Box 18.1   The autonomic nervous system

Sympathetic nerve effects	Parasympathetic nerve effects
Dilate bronchi	Return bronchi to normal diameter
Increase heart rate	Decrease heart rate
Widen pupils	Constrict pupils
Constrict sphincter muscles	Relax sphincter muscles
Dilate or constrict blood vessels	Normalize blood vessel diameter

In other words, the sympathetic system makes it easier to breathe, allows for better circulation and thus oxygenation, brings more light in for better vision, prevents unwanted digestion or elimination of ingested materials, and allows for either smooth blood flow (dilate) or higher blood pressure (constrict). The parasympathetic system generally has the opposite effect.

Clinical case resolution: A puppy dragging one limb

Unfortunately, the person who took blood from the animal used a tourniquet without being properly trained to use one. Application of excessive pressure can cause damage to the nearby nerves (in this case, the radial nerve) and left this puppy with a permanent defect.

Review questions

1   What is cerebellar hypoplasia?
2   What is the resting voltage of the mammalian neuron?
3   What does a node of Ranvier have to do with the transmission of an axon potential?
4   Depolarization of a neuron means that
    _____
5   What is a synapse?
6   What would happen if the neurotransmitter were to stay in the synapse after it has contacted the receptor?
7   What is the difference between a ligand-gated and a voltage-gated channel?
8   What effect does the sympathetic nervous system have on heart rate and respiratory rate?
9   What constitutes the CNS?
10 What is the myotactic reflex?

Chapter **19** Renal Physiology

Clinical case: 12-year-old cat

A client brings in her 12-year-old cat. The cat has been in excellent health until the past couple of months but has recently been showing decreased appetite and activity. He has lost weight and has been grooming himself less than usual. He has been drinking a great deal of water. You tell the client as you are doing the examination that the cat appears dehydrated. She cannot understand how that could be, given that the cat has been taking in so much liquid.

Introduction

All of the blood in the body, at some point, circulates through the kidney. This emphasizes the great importance of the kidney in the maintenance of homeostasis within the organism. What happens when the blood enters the system is the subject of this chapter.

The renal artery enters the kidney at the hilus, and its branches head toward the cortex. The glomerulus of each nephron is within the cortex of the renal parenchyma; in contrast, the tubules of the nephron travel between the glomerulus and the medulla before finally descending through the medulla toward the renal pelvis.

The glomerulus is composed of a tuft of capillaries. As the blood enters the glomerulus, it is filtered through these capillaries. As they are fenestrated, it is easy to see how material can escape into the surrounding areas, with other materials proceeding through. Blood that is not sent along into the systemic circulation continues through to the rest of the nephron. The first of the sections of tubules is the proximal collecting tubule.

The nephron

The nephron as a whole conserves low molecular weight proteins, water, and electrolytes. The glomerulus, in particular, filters out things as large as cells and proteins (especially albumin) so they are not excreted. Other materials are sent back into the body at other points along the system. For example, glucose is "rejected" by the proximal tubules. What passes from the glomerulus into the tubules is known as the glomerular filtrate. As its larger molecules have been filtered away, it actually has almost the same specific gravity as blood plasma (see Figure 19.1).

Anatomy and Physiology for Veterinary Technicians and Nurses: A Clinical Approach, First Edition. Robin Sturtz and Lori Asprea.
© 2012 John Wiley & Sons, Inc. Published 2012 by John Wiley & Sons, Inc.

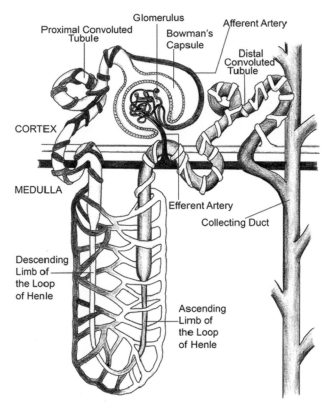

Figure 19.1   The nephron, the basic working unit of the kidney. Cats have fewer of these per kidney than any other mammal.

Clinically, this is quite important. If the specific gravity of the urine (which is, after all, the eventual product of all the filtering the nephrons do) is no different from that of plasma, the nephron has not done its job. One indicator of renal disease is isosthenuria, which is when the specific gravity (molecular "thickness," relative to water) of urine is like that of the glomerular filtrate. If the urine is isosthenuric, almost nothing has happened to it from the time it entered the tubules—which is to say that the tubules are not functional.

The glomerular capillaries are fenestrated, allowing material to be funneled into the tubules. The speed (and, by extension, efficiency) with which this transfer occurs is known as glomerular filtration rate (GFR). There are many factors that determine GFR, which will be discussed below. For the moment, keep in mind that the liters of fluid that pass through the glomerular capillaries will be filtered to a greater or lesser extent. The nature of this filtering is a life-or-death function for mammals.

The glomerular capillaries sit in an epithelial nest called Bowman's capsule. The space the fluid crosses in going from the glomerulus into the first of the tubules is known as Bowman's space. The filtrate crosses that space into the proximal tubule, the first part of the tubular section of the nephron. The majority of fluid that is resorbed from the kidney and sent back into the body comes out of this proximal tubule. There are a few mechanisms that encourage the movement of fluids and proteins back into the body. Among those mechanisms are passive transport and cotransport. Passive transport occurs when material is drawn from one area to another (in this case, from the tubule to the surrounding tissue) by differences in local fluid and tissue pressure. Proteins often are carried by molecules such as sodium and hydrogen (cotransport). Note that glucose, a very large molecule, will be rejected from the proximal tubule and sent back to the body. It is normally the case that all the glucose, which is so crucial for energy production, is sent back to the body. It is only when glucose levels in the bloodstream are very high that glucose overcomes the ability of the glomerulus and tubule to reject it, and it is passed on out of the body in the urine. The combination of hyperglycemia (high blood level of glucose) and glucosuria (glucose in the urine) is the major indicator of diabetes mellitus, a common metabolic disease in dogs and cats (and in humans, for that matter). When we speak of the "renal threshold" for glucose, we refer to that level at which blood glucose levels are so high that not all of it can be resorbed by the kidney. In this case, it will move out of the body in urine.

Active transport also plays a role in moving needed material out of the proximal tubule. Much of this type of transport is accomplished via the Na-K-ATPase pump. As sodium and potassium exchange places, powered by the "energy molecule" ATP, other electrolytes are dragged along as well (e.g., calcium and chloride).

The proximal tubule leads into the loop of Henle, which has ascending and descending parts, referred to as the ascending and descending limb. From the loop of Henle, the filtrate enters the distal convoluted tubule and then the collecting duct. A given collecting duct receives material from more than one nephron.

As important as it is that materials that the body needs are resorbed, it is also crucial that materials that the body should not keep continues through the nephron until it is excreted in the urine. This applies to materials like antibiotics and other drugs, as well as metabolic waste products.

Knowing how antibiotics are processed is particularly important. For example, if a particular antibiotic is mostly filtered out of the body through the kidney, and the kidney is malfunctioning, it is possible that too much of the drug will remain within the system. Knowing an animal's general health is thus particularly important in prescribing medications. Another medication that is, say, broken down elsewhere in the body might be preferable in a case like this.

Renal excretion/resorption of water

Water tends to follow sodium, so resorption of sodium means that water is also being resorbed. Excreting large amounts of sodium means that more water will exit the body. Clearly, loss of too much water is dangerous to most body systems. As a result, not all of the nephron allows water to leave the system. For example, the thick ascending loop of Henle and the distal convoluted tubule (the next section in the nephron) are impermeable to water. Even if sodium is resorbed, water won't follow it.

Permeability to water is not a static thing. Certain hormones affect the nephron's permeability to water. Aldosterone (produced by the adrenal gland) and vasopressin (produced in the pituitary gland) alter how water is exchanged in the nephron and can cause the system to retain more water than it would otherwise.

Aldosterone has a significant effect on the collecting duct as far as the excretion of sodium and the retention of potassium are concerned. The hormones parathormone (PTH) and calcitonin act on the distal parts of the nephron to mediate calcium excretion.

The excretion of urea is another key element in pulling water out of the body or keeping it within the body. Urea is produced in the liver and excreted mostly by the kidney in mammals. Like sodium, it "pulls" water along with it. High levels of urea, which does not generally get resorbed, are kept within the nephron. This favors the excretion of water as it follows urea and sodium out of the body. When urine contains a great deal of water content, it is said to be dilute. It will have a pale color and will be of low specific gravity. If, on the other hand, the nephron resorbs most of the fluid, the remaining urine will be concentrated. Concentrated urine has a dark color and a high specific gravity. It has less water and more materials like proteins and sediment. If there is at least some concentration or dilution of urine, this is an indication of at least some degree of renal function, whether normal or not.

Another factor in the nature of filtrate traveling through the nephron is the countercurrent mechanism. The descending and ascending limbs of the loop of Henle run right next to each other. The descending limb has a tendency to pick up solutes that need to be excreted, and the ascending limb picks up more water. The relative amount of material surrounding the loop varies because of this. That variation creates more or less oncotic pressure and contributes in large measure to how dilute urine becomes.

Having traveled to the distal convoluted tubule and undergone its fluid and solute exchanges, the filtrate moves on to the collecting duct. Here, the Na-K-ATPase pump goes into gear and exchanges electrolytes. From the collecting duct, the material moves toward the renal pelvis. Once the renal filtrate reaches the distal section of the collecting duct and enters the renal pelvis, it is finally referred to as urine.

Water has a great deal to do with systemic blood pressure. If one imagines a garden hose spraying out water, one can understand that having more water in the hose is going to cause the water to spray out faster, as will narrowing the opening through which it exits. The faster the water comes out, the higher the pressure of the water.

In addition, water is crucial in its role as a constituent of cells. Left to its own devices, the glomerulus in a dog or cat would allow dozens of liters of fluid to pass out through the urinary bladder. It is for this reason that the resorption of water in the nephron is such a major function.

Ninety-nine percent of the glomerular filtrate is taken back into the body as it journeys through the nephron. The corollary is that there is always a certain amount of water that is excreted, regardless of how much (or even if) the animal drinks. This is of clinical significance. Even an animal that is not eating or drinking much should still be urinating at least a little, albeit very concentrated urine. An animal in the hospital that is not urinating at all is suffering renal shutdown and needs to be treated as an emergency.

Acid/base balance

The kidney's activities contribute to acid/base balance. One of the characteristics of blood (and urine) is its pH. A low (acidic) pH, associated with high levels of hydrogen ions, can be damaging to body tissues. On the other hand, high levels of bicarbonate are associated with a high pH (alkaline) state. This is not desirable either.

Several systems help regulate the body's acid/base balance, including the respiratory system. The latter contributes by removing more or less CO_2 from the body. Removing large amounts of CO_2 helps raise blood pH. It is for this reason (among others) that hypoxemic animals often pant; the body is trying to raise the pH of the blood as it brings in more oxygen.

The kidney plays a role in this as well. Particularly in the proximal tubule and collecting duct, the nephron can either retain hydrogen ions or excrete them. Part of the series of exchanges of molecules involves bicarbonate (an alkaline molecule) and ammonium ion. The latter is actually produced within the proximal tubule. The eventual outcome of these functions is that in cases of acidosis (pH levels that are too low), bicarbonate is resorbed and hydrogen ion is excreted. This helps raise blood pH.

Blood pressure and the renal system

The control of systemic blood pressure is also in part a function of the kidney. The renin–angiotensin–aldosterone (RAA) system helps control GFR and water resorption. When systemic blood pressure is low, the release of the hormone renin is triggered. Renin comes from cells located near the glomerular capillaries (juxtaglomerular cells). Renin, in turn, stimulates the eventual conversion of a compound called angiotensin I to angiotensin II. Angiotensin I is produced by way of a liver enzyme, and the conversion to angiotensin II is catalyzed by angiotensin-converting enzyme (ACE). The use of many medications that control systemic blood pressure is based on this series of reactions.

The end result of all of these functions is related to angiotensin II. It is a vasoconstrictor, stimulating a decreased venous diameter in order to build blood pressure back up. In addition, it stimulates the adrenal gland to produce aldosterone. Aldosterone, as noted before, affects the collecting duct. It does this by way of pulling sodium and water back into the body. This also helps increase blood pressure.

Further, the level of angiotensin II in the bloodstream is a signal to the pituitary gland to release vasopressin (also known as antidiuretic hormone [ADH]). This increases water resorption in the nephron (among other things) and raises blood pressure.

Of course, if these cycles continued indefinitely, systemic blood pressure would rise too high. To avoid this, a negative feedback loop is built into the system. When plasma levels of angiotensin II reach a certain level, the production of renin is suppressed. This brings the cycle of hormones and enzymes to a halt.

Anemia and the kidney

Another renal hormone is erythropoietin (EPO). This hormone is released in response to a low level of erythrocytes in blood entering the glomerulus. EPO travels to the bone marrow and stimulates red blood cell production. This is of clinical importance. In animals with severe kidney disease, EPO production is affected, and the patient can become anemic. The anemia can be quite severe, in which case we can offer a synthetic EPO in injectable form. It has both advantages and disadvantages, like any drug, and its use is an issue that should be discussed with any client whose pet is suffering from renal malfunction.

A note about bilirubin should be made. Bilirubin is a constituent of red blood cells. In the liver, it is converted to urobilinogen, which is partly excreted in the feces. Some of it undergoes conversion in the bloodstream and is excreted in urine. In fact, it contributes to the yellow color of urine. There should not be intact bilirubin in urine. If there is, renal and/or circulatory and/or hepatic disease should be investigated.

Species differences

Avians have three renal arteries. They also have no loop of Henle in the nephron. Most of the salt resorption in their system is achieved in the gastrointestinal (GI) tract. The GI and urinary excreta are channeled to the same exit point, the cloaca. Note that avians excrete urea crystals, and there is little or no liquid urine eliminated by a healthy animal.

Clinical case resolution: 12-year-old cat

In the case described at the start of this chapter, we were presented with a cat with chronic renal disease. When the nephron is malfunctioning, its ability to either conserve or excrete water is hampered. Since it can do neither, it simply lets almost all of the fluid flow through, without resorbing any of it. The central nervous system assumes the animal needs to drink more as he is urinating away so much liquid. Thus begins a cycle of drinking and urinating in increasing amounts, while none of the fluid is actually being used to hydrate the animal. This is a common problem and is usually solved by giving the animal fluids subcutaneously so that they can be absorbed directly by the tissues.

Review questions

1 Name the parts of the nephron, starting with where it receives blood from the arterioles.
2 What can be inferred about the function of the nephron if the urine matches the glomerular filtrate?
3 True or false: All parts of the nephron are permeable to water.
4 Renal failure can be associated with anemia. Why?
5 What does aldosterone do to the nephron?
6 True or false: As water is being absorbed or excreted by the nephron, it will tend to follow absorption or excretion of calcium but not sodium.
7 True or false: An animal that has not had anything to drink all day will still urinate.

Chapter **20** Cardiovascular Physiology

Clinical case: German shepherd with dilated cardiomyopathy

In completing a physical examination of a German Shepherd with dilated cardiomyopathy (an enlargement of the heart), the veterinarian simultaneously auscults the heart and places two fingers over the femoral artery to check the pulse. The veterinarian explains that she is checking for a pulse deficit. The following chapter will help explain why she is doing this.

Introduction

Conventionally, discussion of the circulatory system begins with the heart. As the primary muscle controlling the movement of blood throughout the body, it is the key player in distributing blood and its contents throughout the system. The continued pumping of the heart is associated with the living animal; indeed, the methods of euthanasia we commonly employ indirectly or directly involve the circulatory system.

The heartbeat

The heart generates its own action potential, allowing it to maintain direct control over its function to a large degree. The pacemaker cells are those that initiate the impulse. They are situated in the wall of the right atrium, just as the vena cava enters the chamber. These cells form a structure called the sinoatrial (SA) node (see Figure 20.1).

The depolarization of the node generates an electrical impulse that flows to the left and right atria, inciting a change in the muscle fibers that ultimately causes them to contract. As a result of the branching structure of the muscle fibers, and the connections between them called gap junctions, the muscle fibers are able to fire in concert. This lends strength to the muscle movement.

There are fibers that also conduct the depolarizing wave from the SA node to an area near the atrial septum, where the atrium and the ventricles meet. This area is called the atrioventricular (AV) node. From the AV node, the wave of electrical energy continues through a "cable" of cells called the bundle of His.

The wave of energy then separates into two sections. They are called the left branch bundle and the right branch bundle. These

Anatomy and Physiology for Veterinary Technicians and Nurses: A Clinical Approach, First Edition. Robin Sturtz and Lori Asprea.
© 2012 John Wiley & Sons, Inc. Published 2012 by John Wiley & Sons, Inc.

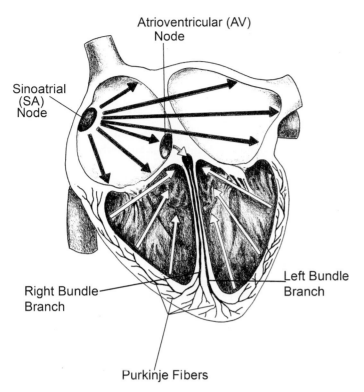

Atrioventricular (AV)
Node

Sinoatrial
(SA)
Node

Left Bundle
Branch

Right Bundle
Branch

Purkinje Fibers

Figure 20.1   The direct control of the heartbeat arises from the sinoatrial node. The signal travels from there to the atrioventricular node and onward along the ventricular septum toward each side of the heart.

cells transmit the energy down along the ventricular septum. When they reach the apex of the heart, they split off and go along the myocardial wall of each ventricle, climbing up the wall of the left and right ventricle back toward the base of the heart.

The bundles are composed of something called Purkinje fibers. These are the support structure of the cells carrying the electrical energy that is being transmitted to the muscle fibers. It is important to note that this transmission is carried by cells, not nerve fibers. In other words, the internal changes in the electrical charge within the cells of the heart that lead to muscle contraction are spread by cells and soft tissue, not by nerves. As noted in the chapter regarding muscle function (Chapter 16), the autonomic nervous system does have some input to the heartbeat, but the heart itself generates direct control over its movements.

The impulse actually slows down as it crosses the AV node. This plays a crucial role in the generation of the heartbeat. Slowing the energy wave down allows it to gather itself together and generate a strong, organized "push" so that the ventricles contract as a whole.

One of the unique features of this system is that it is possible for cells anywhere along the route of the depolarization wave to initiate the electrical energy change; that is, the SA node is not the only place that the heartbeat can be triggered. By the same token, if the electrical stimulus is generated further down the system, it will not necessarily be transmitted in as organized a fashion. This has significant import for diagnosing heart disease.

If the pacemaker cells are not firing in a synchronous manner, the heartbeat will be irregular. It may "skip" a beat, or beat less efficiently. An irregular heartbeat can be a direct result of irregular/disorganized transmission of the electrical wave that stimulates the heart muscle.

As is true in the neurological system, the transmission of energy within the pacemaker cells and from them to the muscle fibers relies in large measure on the electrolytes sodium, calcium, and potassium. Abnormalities in any one of these can have serious consequences for the function of the heart. In fact, when we mentioned euthanasia at the beginning of this chapter, what we were referring to was the fact that a large amount of potassium will disrupt the system to the point where the hearbeat stops altogether. Without the ability to pump blood (and thus oxygen) to the cells, death of the animal results.

One other note concerns the metabolism of the muscle fibers within the heart. We mentioned several ways that skeletal muscle fibers generate energy. In contrast, the heart specifically uses cellular respiration to generate ATP. It makes very little use of carbohydrate derivatives. Therefore, oxygen is particularly crucial to heart function, more so than to skeletal muscle.

Cardiac output

A number of factors are involved in the heartbeat. The electrical energy that sparks the initial muscle contraction is only a part of the picture. For example, part of what determines how much blood is pumped out of the heart is related to the rate at which the heart beats. The amount of blood pumped out of the heart in one beat is called stroke volume. Multiplying that number by the speed of the heartbeats, or heart rate, yields a number that is referred to as cardiac output. Cardiac output is the reflection of the amount of blood sent out to the body over a period of time. Any change in stroke volume or heart rate will affect cardiac output.

Stroke volume can be affected by a number of factors. These include level of exercise, general health of the animal's heart, systemic blood pressure, and the autonomic nervous system. If systemic blood pressure is high, for example, the heart has to beat harder. This will increase stroke volume. Eventually, the abnormal strain on the heart will damage it, and stroke volume will actually decrease, leading to a decrease in cardiac output.

Enlargement of the heart muscle causes abnormalities in the heart rate. As is true for any muscle, the harder it works, the larger it will grow, and the more rapid the heart rate needed to keep up the pace. If the heart is too big, it will no longer beat in an organized fashion.

There are genetic factors in some animals that affect cardiac output. Certain breeds of dogs are prone to something called dilated cardiomyopathy; some cat breeds have a very high incidence of genetically based hypertrophic cardiomyopathy. The terms dilated and hypertrophic refer to patterns of muscle enlargement. The separate terms refer to the exact nature of the structural abnormality in the tissue. In either case, the enlargement causes a number of problems, including the inability of the heart to sustain normal cardiac output. In dogs, breeds affected include Doberman pinschers and German Shepherds. In cats, Maine coons and Norwegian Forest cats suffer from heart disease much more commonly than in domestic shorthair cats.

The pressure in the ventricle as blood is about to flow into it is known as preload. Preload is essentially the degree to which the ventricles match the pressure in the atria during diastole (the part of the heartbeat during which the valves between atrium and ventricle are open). The ventricles eventually reach a point where they are filled. At that point, the ventricles will expel the blood out of the heart by contracting, called systole. Preload can be thought of as the amount of tension the ventricles have to match in order to efficiently pump blood out of the heart.

As might be expected, the greater the pressure/blood content in the ventricles, the stronger the force of the blood that is pushed out of them (e.g., into the aorta). The relationship between the preload and the stroke volume is described by Starling's law. As a result of this relationship, the more blood in the ventricle when it is filled, the greater the stroke volume will be.

This does not seem to be a remarkable statement, but it has tremendous import for the circulatory system. For example, if stroke volume increases on one side of the heart, by Starling's law, the other side will try to match it so that the amount of blood remains constant. As a clinical example, the presence of heartworms in the pulmonary artery will cause an increase in pressure in the right atrium (the chamber from which blood comes into the pulmonary artery). Unfortunately, the pulmonary artery is where uncontrolled heartworm infestation often settles. This increase in pressure will be reflected in increased preload and, thus, increased cardiac output.

Another factor affecting cardiac output is the contractility of the heart muscle. The stronger the heart muscle's contraction, the more blood can be expelled. Both the sympathetic nervous system and certain medications can increase contractility. If the heart muscle cannot contract enough to produce a strong burst of energy, not all of the blood can be expelled from the ventricle. In other words, stroke volume decreases.

One of the ways that systemic blood pressure is kept at a normal level is by maintaining normal cardiac output. Less blood entering the peripheral circulation means less fluid pressure, which means that the flow of blood throughout the body will be less efficient, and oxygenation of body tissues will be compromised. The types of heart enlargement mentioned above also affect contractility.

There is also a phenomenon called afterload. If pressure in the aorta is very high, it will impede the attempt of the ventricle to empty completely. Small increases in afterload generally can be overcome by the healthy heart, but in cases of heart disease, it can become a significant impairment.

The circulatory system can be thought of as two circuits. One goes from the heart to the lungs and back to the heart, and can be referred to as the pulmonary circuit. The other goes from the heart to the rest of the body and then back again. The circulation throughout the body is referred to as peripheral, or systemic, circulation. Please refer to the chapter on circulatory anatomy to recall the vessels involved in the flow of blood through the body. For the moment, think of the circulation of blood from the heart

as traveling through the arteries, narrowing as they approach the capillaries, and then from the capillaries through veins that widen as they approach the cranial and caudal vena cava, which return the blood to the heart.

Flow through the heart and back

Blood flowing back from the body toward the heart travels through venules and veins until it reaches either the cranial or caudal vena cava. They merge and enter the heart at the right atrium. Therefore, all systemic circulation leads back to the right atrium of the heart. As the atrium fills, the right AV valve will open. At this point, the atrium contracts, and the blood is forced through the opening into the right ventricle. When the right ventricle has filled sufficiently, the right AV valve snaps shut and the semilunar valve of the pulmonary trunk will open. The pulmonary trunk is an artery in that blood is flowing away from the heart. It does not carry oxygenated blood, unlike other arteries. In fact, the destination of blood from the pulmonary trunk is the lungs, where oxygen and carbon dioxide will be exchanged.

The oxygenated blood is carried toward the heart in the pulmonary veins. There are two or three in dogs and cats, and they lead directly into the left atrium. As it fills, the left AV (mitral) valve will open, and blood will enter the left ventricle. When full enough, the mitral valve closes, and the contraction of the heart pushes the blood through the semilunar valve that guards the entrance to the aorta.

Note that the left and right AV valves open and close at the same time. In other words, blood flows from the atrium to the ventricle on each side of the heart at the same moment. Similarly, the contraction of the ventricles that sends blood to the lung or the rest of the body (i.e., to the pulmonary trunk or the aorta) occurs at one time.

When blood fills the ventricles, a signal is triggered by the increase in fluid pressure that causes the AV valves to snap shut. At this point, the semilunar valves of the aorta and pulmonary artery open and the ventricles contract. This strong contraction is called systole. Systole exerts the maximum pressure from the heart on the arteries. Once most of the blood has been expelled from the ventricles, the AV valves open and the semilunar valves close, and the cycle repeats. The contraction of the atria then sends blood into the ventricles. This contraction is referred to as diastole.

Clinical measurement of the strength of the diastolic and systolic contraction is usually done indirectly, using the measure of systemic blood pressure as an indicator. We refer to diastolic and systolic pressure. As the atria are smaller and are sending blood a relatively short distance, the resting pressure inside the atria is much lower than that inside the ventricles. Therefore, the diastolic number should also be smaller than the systolic number when measuring the strength of the contraction. When an animal's blood pressure is reported as, say, 90/150 (ninety over one-fifty), we are comparing the relative strength of the diastolic to the systolic heart contraction.

As might be imagined, the transmission of force as the blood circulates will diminish as the blood goes further away from the heart. The aorta is the largest in diameter of all the arteries and is composed mainly of elastic tissue. This reflects the fact that the full force of the systolic pressure is accepted by this vessel. In fact, one of the reasons that many arteries, particularly those nearest the heart, follow a circuitous route relates to an attempt to dampen some of this great force as the blood enters the smaller (narrower) blood vessels.

One may also use this to advantage when doing physical examinations. The heartbeat and the pulse of blood through the arteries should be simultaneous. The doctor or the technician will often auscult the heart while feeling for the rhythm of the pulse of the femoral artery. We mentioned in an earlier chapter that the heartbeat and the femoral pulse should be simultaneous. If there is an audible lag between the two, there is some disruption of the circulatory system. This phenomenon is referred to as pulse deficit.

On the subject of auscaulting the heart, it is worthwhile to remember that the dog and cat (as is true in the primate) should have two distinct heart sounds. Each sound is associated with the closing of the AV valves or the semilunar valves; that is, diastole and systole have a sound associated with each. This is not true across all species. For example, the heart of the dog has two sounds, but that of the horse three sounds, when it beats.

A heart murmur reflects turbulence in the flow of blood. Instead of flowing in a single, smooth course from the atrium to the ventricle to the body, the blood may reach a structural abnormality that causes a whirlpool or some other swirling affect. Sometimes, the valves are abnormal and do not close completely. This allows blood to stream backward instead of forward. It is common in older, small-breed dogs to find abnormalities in the mitral valve. The valve is often thickened or deformed and does not close all the way. Thus, blood travels backward through the small opening from the ventricle, back into the atrium. This produces a swishing sound.

There are causes of heart murmurs that are not from primary heart disease. For example, anemia can be associated with turbulent blood flow. Hyperthyroidism can also cause heart murmurs; the high level of activity of the gland forces the blood to swirl as it travels through the heart.

As blood is expelled into the aorta, there are a series of vessels called cardiac arteries that branch off to bring fresh blood to supply the heart itself with oxygen. It is crucial to the rest of the body that the heart be in good working order. Thus, it is no surprise that the most highly oxygenated blood goes to the heart muscle first.

Recall that there is a greater or lesser degree of muscle tissue in the lining of the arteries. Making the arteries narrower increases the pressure of the blood flowing through it. While this is efficient in speeding the blood along to where it is needed, it also means that the force involved can, over the long term, damage the vessels themselves. The narrowing and dilation of blood vessels is accomplished by the smooth muscle in the lining of the vessels, mediated by the autonomic nervous system. The greatest control is actually in the arterioles. Some of them actually have sphincter muscles that can narrow these vessels tremendously, allowing pressure to build up. In contrast, the venules

have no muscle tissue as their acceptance of blood returning to the heart is passive.

As arteries reach the outskirts of their travels, they have not only narrowed in diameter but have also undergone physical changes. There is less elastic tissue and more muscle tissue in arterioles than in the aorta and in some of the other major vessels. This will come into play as we discuss the control of blood pressure.

Eventually, the arterioles reach the capillaries, which are the smallest blood vessels. Their diameter is usually less than $10\,\mu m$. This fact, in addition to the presence of small pores in the walls of the capillaries, allows material to be exchanged with the tissue surrounding the vessels.

A combination of diffusion and hydrostatic pressure helps determine what materials are absorbed by the surrounding tissue and what materials are resorbed by the capillaries to continue through the venous system back to the heart.

Since there is less oxygen in the surrounding tissue than in the artery, the oxygen will flow into the local tissues. The reverse is true for carbon dioxide. Some hormones and lipids can also pass through the pores. All of these materials are conveyed to the cells so that they can use the energy contained therein to produce protein (or whatever else the cell is designed to manufacture).

Hydrostatic pressure has to do with fluid exchange. As the relative water pressure is higher within the capillaries than in the surrounding area, water tends to flow out of the capillaries to hydrate the tissues. Changes in the normal balance of these pressures, as might be the case in dehydration, will lead to an inefficient exchange, exacerbating the water deprivation of the surrounding area by encouraging water to go into the capillaries instead.

As noted in Chapter 8, the capillaries in certain areas, such as the liver and the kidney, are fenestrated. They have large pores that allow bigger molecules (like proteins) to flow into and out of the capillaries. In the liver, where toxins are processed, it is desirable to having a way to "flush" them directly into the liver from the circulatory system.

Blood pressure

The mere act of flowing through the blood vessels means that the blood will be affected by the stiffness or natural pressure within the vessel itself. The resistance of the circulatory system is analogous to a person walking into the wind. Under normal circumstances, the resistance is the equivalent of a light breeze; in disease states, or under "deliberate" increases in resistance caused by the hormonal and/or neurological system, it is more like walking into a storm.

The combination of the cardiac output and the resistance of the peripheral vasculature determines arterial pressure. Note that there is also resistance in the veins. The greatest resistance to blood flow is actually in the arterioles. The fierce pumping of the blood provided by the heart propels the blood through the arteries. This, combined with the structure of the arterial wall, means that the blood should flow under a certain amount of pressure as it travels toward the organs and other tissues. As it reaches the smaller-diameter vessels such as the arterioles, the blood is flowing under higher pressure.

This is clearly advantageous. Any disease states that lower the cardiac output, or weaken the stiffness of the arteries, will have a negative effect on the ability of blood to circulate. Arterial stiffness in animals, unlike in humans, is actually rare. Changes in cardiac output, however, do occur. Note that certain drugs lower cardiac output; when using these drugs or anesthetics, it is important to measure systemic blood pressure carefully.

When the animal is exercising, the arterioles in the skeletal muscles actually expand. This means that they can accept a much greater volume of blood. This explains (in part) how the animal can cope with the greater activity required during exercise. It also explains why the animal suffers from exercise intolerance with significant cardiac disease.

Note also that the blood vessels within the lung are quite sensitive to the amount of oxygen within the blood. In cases of oxygen deprivation, their diameter will be adjusted, lowering their resistance and allowing more blood to flow, and exchange more carbon dioxide for oxygen.

Cardiac output is affected by contractility and heart rate. Other factors also control the resistance of the arterioles, increasing or decreasing blood pressure. Factors such as neurological input, hormones, and/or the condition of the destination tissues also have an effect.

Autonomic nervous system involvement

The autonomic nervous system controls both the function of the heart itself and the degree of constriction of the arteries and veins. The sympathetic nervous system uses epinephrine and norepinephrine as transmitters to increase the rate of impulses through the pacemaker cells and to increase the strength of the cardiac muscle contraction. The parasympathetic system, by way of acetylcholine, has the opposite effect.

The sympathetic nerve fibers control the peripheral arterioles and veins by two methods. One is the constriction of the arterioles and veins. There is one class of sympathetic nerve receptor cells that actually causes vasodilation. These receptors are present in the coronary arteries and in skeletal muscles. Dilation of these vessels allows more oxygen-carrying blood to reach these tissues.

The parasympathetic fibers in the heart stimulate muscarinic cholinergic receptors that slow its rate and, thus, cardiac output. Muscarinic receptors are also present in the arterioles, and their stimulation causes vasodilation.

Hormonal influence is a subset of neurological input, as the release of hormones such as epinephrine and norepinephrine is mediated by the sympathetic nervous system. However, the increase in production of these hormones (used as neurotransmitters) is not possible without the function of the adrenal gland, so the endocrine system is crucial to the control of blood pressure.

Specialized cells within the local organs and tissues also contribute to influence over blood flow. Baroreceptors are pressure-sensitive nerve fibers. When arterial pressure goes above or below its desired amount, the change in pressure within the vessel is sensed by these cells. It is actually the stretching of the walls of the surrounding tissue that triggers the response. What is engendered is an increase in the number of action potentials over time. The neural impulse is directed to the hypothalamus.

This message will result in the autonomic nervous system adjusting cardiac output and vascular resistance to counteract the undesired changes. Baroreceptor cells are located in the aortic arch, the right atrium of the heart, and the carotid arteries. Note that these adjustments do not necessarily bring the systemic blood pressure all the way back to normal. In addition, they do not address the source of the disturbance; they merely alert the brain to the problem.

There are also stretch receptors within the atria. These respond to the volume of blood present. They work in concert with the baroreceptor cells to speed up or decrease the frequency of the action potentials sent to the central nervous system.

There are other mechanisms related to the outside world that mediate vascular circulation. For example, the "fight or flight" response is triggered by the perception of stimuli perceived as threatening. The central nervous system's interpretation of any menacing event (including everything from a loud noise to a leaping tiger) will set off the release of hormones such as vasopressin and angiotensin II in response to the sympathetic nervous system's engagement. Certainly, the cardiovascular system will respond with increased cardiac output and systemic blood pressure. Anyone who has ausculted the chest of a timid cat in the clinic is well aware of this phenomenon.

The mechanism works in the opposite way as well. As the animal's activity slows, the parasympathetic system becomes more active (and the sympathetic system less so). This allows for the "rest and digest" state, in which case the cardiac output and systemic blood pressure will return to its resting level. Sleep, of course, is a strong expression of this change.

If blood pressure becomes low enough, and the cardiac output and vascular system do not compensate, the animal can undergo syncope (fainting). This is rare in animals, although not uncommon in humans. Again, animals receiving treatment or medication that lowers blood pressure must be monitored carefully. Syncope or decreased consciousness may be a sign that there has been an overdose of the medication.

Measurement of systemic blood pressure is usually accomplished indirectly, by way of monitoring the strength of the pulse through a systemic artery. As with measuring core temperature by way of a thermometer placed away from the major organs, the measurement of blood pressure using a distal artery yields a slightly different result from that which would be found measuring these levels closer to the heart.

The lymphatic system

Blood and other molecules along for the ride travel from the capillaries through the venous system. The majority of the veins actually have a larger diameter than that of the arteries (the aorta being a notable exception). Thus, the venous system can actually carry a large percentage of blood volume.

Along the way, lymphatic vessels exit from the organs and other structures. These vessels have the ability to draw off larger molecules, like plasma proteins and fragments of dead cells. These vessels travel throughout the body, just as blood vessels do, although they are lesser in number.

The lymph nodes perform a valuable filtering service. The white blood cells they contain have the ability to destroy pathogens such as bacteria. Cells called macrophages can scavenge unwanted material and "digest" it so that it ceases to be a threat to the system.

The lymph nodes assist in the storage of white blood cells as well, which can then be sent out into the system to respond to inflammation. Materials that have been processed in the lymph node are then funneled into the efferent vessels toward the veins, usually the vena cava. Thus, the venous system not only carries blood cells back to the heart for diversion to the lungs to pick up oxygen. It also provides a way for the disposal of filtered lymphatic fluid.

Clinical case resolution: German shepherd with dilated cardiomyopathy

The strong pulse of blood through the arteries has its origins, as we have seen, in the heart. The wave of pulsation should be almost simultaneous with the heartbeat. If the pulse in the femoral artery is not synchronous with that of the heart, there is clearly some abnormality in the vessels or the cardiac output that causes this. The deep femoral artery is used for this monitoring in dogs and cats because it normally has an easily distinguishable beat and because it is readily accessible for palpation.

Review questions

1 Define cardiac output.
2 What would happen if a heartbeat was triggered by the AV node rather than the SA node?
3 Define Starling's law.
4 The term systole refers to simultaneous contraction of the _____ of the heart.
5 Increased pressure or valve stiffness in the aorta can increase its resistance to blood flow. This resistance is referred to as _____.
6 The baroreceptors respond to _____.
7 Define pulse deficit.
8 What is the effect of increasing the diameter of the blood vessels on blood pressure?
9 Does contractility affect cardiac output?
10 When lymphatic fluid exits the lymph node, it returns to the circulatory system by way of the arteries or the veins?

Chapter **21** Digestive Physiology

Clinical case: Tarry stool

One of the most common problems encountered in the clinic is the animal with vomiting and/or diarrhea. There are a number of reasons for these symptoms. However, some signs can be specific. A dog coming into the clinic with a poor appetite and dark, tarry feces is identified as having problems related to the stomach or small intestine. While this is not diagnostic of a specific disease, it tells the clinician where to start looking for the problem. How we relate this finding to these parts of the system will become clear during the discussion in this chapter.

Introduction

In Chapter 9, it was noted that the system is extraordinarily complex, both within and among species. In discussing the physiology, the complexity increases. This chapter will concentrate on cats and dogs, with a nod toward other species. The basic function of the digestive tract is to receive, mechanically reduce, and chemically process materials such that nutrients are absorbed and unnecessary materials are excreted. Nutrients are absorbed so that they can be directed to the rest of the body by way of the bloodstream. Feces are the materials excreted from the digestive tract. While the renal system also excretes material, it has a completely different biochemical function and so is treated as a completely separate entity.

The entryway

Any material the animal ingests that preserves life is considered a nutrient. This includes things that may not be considered as food by the layperson.

In critical nursing, one of the first considerations is hydration status. Water is not only a nutrient, but it is also one of the most important ones. Animals can live longer without food than without water. As noted earlier, much of the composition of the cells of the body is water. The accessibility of potable water is crucial, and the ability to drink it essential.

In dogs and cats, most food is accessed by a combination of the lips, tongue, and teeth. Food can be brought in by lips,

Anatomy and Physiology for Veterinary Technicians and Nurses: A Clinical Approach, First Edition. Robin Sturtz and Lori Asprea.
© 2012 John Wiley & Sons, Inc. Published 2012 by John Wiley & Sons, Inc.

tongue, and teeth to varying degrees, depending on the nature of the food. In horses, the lips are prehensile; they are very mobile, and can actually wrap around grasses in order to bring them into the mouth, almost like an elephant's trunk.

Once inside the mouth, a number of activities begin. Mechanical digestion, which is to say the physical grinding down of the food, is accomplished by grinding of the teeth and movement of the bolus (literally, ball) of food by the tongue and buccinator (cheek) muscles so that material is shifted from one side of the mouth to the other. This would be difficult if the material were dry. The salivary glands are stimulated by the smell and/or feel of food in the mouth. They produce saliva, which, in addition to moisture, has small amounts of enzymes that aid in digestion. For example, canine saliva contains some amylase, which helps digest starches. There is little, if any, amylase in feline saliva. This is not surprising, considering that felines are true carnivores, while canines are omnivores. Felines thus have much less starch in their diet (at least, they should).

Note that the mouth has functions other than those of digestion. The mouth has a role in amplifying sound. It also serves a respiratory function, allowing air to pass in and out when the nasal passages are not able to conduct enough air during breathing. The mucous membranes of the mouth help in thermoregulation in that their moisture allows for the evaporation that aids in cooling when the mouth is open. Finally, the teeth serve as a method of defense or aggression (or both).

Teeth

The term "hypsodont" refers to teeth that continue to grow throughout the animals' life. Dog and cat teeth are not hypsodont. In dogs and cats, the "puppy" or "kitty" teeth that grow during the first few months of life are referred to as deciduous, meaning temporary, teeth. The adult teeth start to grow underneath them, and eventually the deciduous teeth are pushed out of the mouth and the adult teeth remain. The adult, or permanent, teeth in dogs and cats stay the same size for the rest of the animals' lives.

However, in horses, the teeth continue to increase in length and thickness as the animal ages. Only the acts of chewing and food abrasion keep the teeth from growing too big. In rabbits, the incisor teeth are also hypsodont.

Dental care is important in all animals. Diseases of the teeth and gums can be associated with problems in many organ systems, particularly in the gastrointestinal (GI) tract and heart. Since equine teeth can easily overgrow, particularly if the animal's diet is inappropriate or if there is an abnormal chewing pattern, regular dental care is crucial. The abnormal size and shape of teeth under these conditions can cause pain and even reluctance to eat. Filing the teeth down to a normal size and shape is called "floating" the teeth.

Neglected rabbits can have such severe overgrowth of the maxillary incisors that they are unable to eat; the teeth can curve over the lower teeth and start to curl toward the chin. Most often, a Dremel drill is used to bring the teeth down to a normal size. The same procedure is used to trim the beak of a bird. A rabbit whose teeth are severely overgrown will sometimes have to have part of the crown of the tooth cut off by a clipper-type instrument called a rongeur.

The tartar that forms on the teeth of dogs and cats contains bacteria. Left uncleaned, the bacteria can travel throughout the bloodstream and GI tract as they are swallowed. At one time, dental disease was one of the main causes of endocarditis (infection of the heart valves or interior of the cardiac chambers) as some of the bacteria would settle into the nooks and crannies of the valve structure. See Figure 21.1 for a modified Triadan chart. The Triadan system is a way of numbering the teeth so that they can be identified easily. It is more efficient to note that tooth 204 is missing than to say that the maxillary left canine is missing. Using a chart like this, which can be printed onto the dental medical record, makes it easy to record which teeth are missing or extracted when dental work is done.

In dogs and cats, the teeth accomplish both biting and tearing functions. This breaks food into manageable pieces so that it can be swallowed. These pieces are shepherded toward the caudal oral cavity by the tongue. As the bolus of food reaches the caudal oral cavity, the swallow reflex is triggered.

Toward the stomach

Recall that as the oropharynx extends caudally, it divides into two branches. One, the trachea, is designed only to transport air. If food or water were to travel down the trachea, it would access the bronchi and significantly interfere with the function of the lungs. One reason we insist that dogs and cats be fasted before undergoing anesthesia is that if there is food in the upper GI tract and the animal has an emetic reaction to anesthesia (i.e., throws up in reaction to the drug), the food may be aspirated or drawn down the trachea instead of remaining in the esophagus. The epiglottis closes when the animal swallows, and the vocal cords close, in order to prevent this occurrence when the animal is eating.

When eating or drinking, the food ideally follows the path down into the esophagus. A combination of striated and smooth muscles contracts and expands in a rolling wave to push the bolus of food toward the stomach. This wave is referred to as peristalsis.

The initiation of peristalsis sets in motion the production of digestive enzymes in the stomach. As the bolus of food reaches the distal esophagus, its sphincter opens, allowing the food to enter the stomach. If the sphincter were open at all times, food could proceed from the stomach into the esophagus and even exit the body. Some diseases cause reverse peristalsis such that ingesta exit the body. This is known as emesis, better known as vomiting.

While most people use the term GI tract to refer to the entire tube from mouth to anus, GI stands for gastrointestinal. Therefore, properly, GI only refers to the system from the stomach to the exit from the body. It is also important to remember that digestive activity is mostly mediated by the parasympathetic nervous system.

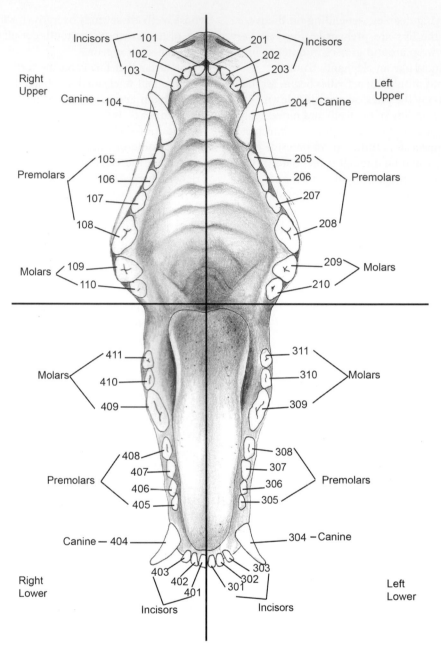

Figure 21.1   The modified Triadan chart is a way of identifying each tooth by a separate number, such that it is clear which teeth are on the left or right, and which are maxillary or mandibular. For numbering purposes, the mouth is divided into four quadrants: upper left, upper right, lower left, and lower right.

The stomach

Once food reaches the stomach, a number of changes occur. The rugae of the stomach are more convoluted and greater in number than the rugae of the dorsal oral cavity. These gastric luminal ridges expand and contract as do the muscles of the stomach wall, and serve to increase the surface area of the stomach. They also help to some extent in mechanically breaking down food.

The luminal surface of the stomach is covered with microscopic goblet cells, which produce mucus. Mucus not only helps lubricate the ingesta (which is what the food and water is now called) but also helps buffer the tissue of the stomach against the low pH of its fluids.

Deep to the mucus-producing cells, and also on a microscopic level, are a series of peaks and valleys. The peaks resemble a finger being pointed and are referred to as villi. Halfway down the villi are parietal cells, which produce hydrochloric acid. At the bottom of the villus, in the "valley," are chief cells, which produce an enzyme called pepsinogen. Pepsinogen leads to the production of pepsin; this transformation is triggered by low pH. Pepsin is particularly important in protein digestion and thus plays a major role in the GI tract of carnivores and omnivores. The goal of antacid medications is to reduce the overproduction of these fluids.

The production of hydrochloric acid (HCl) is helpful in breaking down food products by virtue of its acidic nature. The by-product of HCl production is bicarbonate (HCO_3). Bicarbonate is quite alkaline. As it leaves the cells of the stomach lining and enters the bloodstream, it actually raises the pH of the bloodstream. Thus, the act of acidifying stomach contents actually leads to a high blood pH in carnivores after eating. These fluctuations in pH are also of clinical importance in both evaluating the overall acidity of the system and fashioning drugs to treat various disorders.

A material called gastrin is produced by G cells in the stomach lining (and in the pancreas and duodenum). Gastrin has an effect on parietal cells (and, on a lesser level, chief cells) to produce more HCl and pepsin. As mentioned earlier, the bloodstream undergoes a rising pH as food is digested. Once pH reaches a certain point, a negative feedback loop is triggered regarding gastrin; that is, the higher the pH of the blood, the greater the pressure to decrease gastrin production. In other words, as digestion continues, less gastrin is needed, and so rising pH signals the cells to stop producing gastrin.

Another "side effect" of gastrin production is the release of histamine in the stomach, which also contributes to the eventual lowering of stomach pH. Thus, antihistamines can also play a role in changing gastric pH.

As the enzymes do their work, a number of chemical changes occur, involving the breakdown of nutrients into their constituents. Proteins are broken down into amino acids. Starches are broken down into short-chain polysaccharides.

Entering the intestine

Once the food bolus reaches the pyloric antrum and enzyme activity increases, the pyloric sphincter will open, allowing the ingesta to continue into the duodenum. Once in the duodenum, the ingesta are exposed to enzymes ultimately contributed by the pancreas. These are amylase, lipase, and trypsin.

Amylase is an enzyme that helps digest starches. Lipase, as the root word "lipid" implies, helps digest fats. By the process of elimination, trypsin "digests" proteins.

In discussing the endocrine system, the role of the pancreas as an endocrine organ is noted in that it produces several hormones. Insulin is one of those. The digestive enzymes are not hormones. The production of these enzymes is called exocrine rather than endocrine. Thus, the pancreas is both an exocrine and an endocrine organ. It is the exocrine function that we discuss in connection with digestion.

In addition to providing a place for preliminary digestion of starches, fats, and proteins, the duodenum has a role in entero-hepatic circulation. As is implied by its name, there is a loop between the small intestine (root word "entero-") and liver (hepatic is the adjectival form for liver) that involves the circulation of substances like bile acids. These help the system regulate itself.

When the ingesta reach the duodenum, a signal is sent to the gallbladder telling it to release bile. The bile enters the duodenum by way of a papilla (mound) through which the bile duct discharges its contents. The bile acids are vital for fat digestion. As the acids continue to work, they eventually reach the ileum. At this point, they are broken down enough to circulate back to the liver to suppress bile production. This, too, is a negative feedback loop and another example of the way in which the system is self-sustaining without the animal's conscious control.

Throughout the small intestine, digestive molecules produced in the enterocytes (cells of the small intestine) percolate through the lining of the intestine and are directed out into the lumen of the intestine. This is known as the membranous phase of digestion. There are specific enzymes for the various polysaccharides and peptides (protein products) allowing them to be processed.

Cranially in the GI system, carbohydrates are broken down into lactose, starch, and sucrose. In the membranous phase of digestion, these items are further broken down into various sugars.

Of all of the materials the organism ingests, some are not needed. However, many of them are. It is mostly within the small intestine that material is absorbed to be channeled into systemic circulation. This absorption is accomplished in a number of ways.

Some material passively moves from within the lumen of the intestine to the surrounding tissue and circulation. For example, water is able to "slip out" between cells of the intestinal wall. Passive transport usually is most efficient when the balance of molecular weight favors osmotic movement.

Another method of exchange is called cotransport. The most common example of this involves sodium. An electrolyte crucial to the production of many types of energy, its exit from the intestine can "drag along" other molecules such as glucose. Water is another molecule that tends to follow sodium, described in detail when looking at the function of the nephron in the kidney.

Active transport involves the production of energy that pushes or pulls material into or out of a cell. In the case of the GI tract, it is ATP that, when hydrolyzed, forces sodium out between the cells of the intestinal wall (and allowing potassium in). Recall that hydrolysis is the action of breaking chemical bonds by inserting a water molecule. Hydrolysis is a major player in digestion and is another reason that hydration status is a key part of normal function. It should also be noted that a by-product of hydrolysis is bicarbonate. This contributes to the overall rise in blood pH that accompanies digestion.

The absorption of nutrients is not the only function of digestion. Some materials do need to be excreted; these do not normally transport out of the intestine. (In fact, one of the hallmarks of GI disease is that materials are not absorbed or excreted properly.) For example, if the ingesta has a high salt content, it will actually draw water into the intestine from the surrounding tissue, and thus too much water will be excreted.

The microscopic structure of the jejunum and ileum includes the presence of villi. They are tallest in the jejunum and get shorter and broader as the system continues toward the anus. The enzymes produced in the villi differ from place to place.

The small and large intestines also maintain a wave of peristalsis. Different sections of the bowel are active at any given time, which is why the intestine appears to change shape as the animal is digesting. The term motility refers to the movement of the walls of the digestive tract. We generally refer to intestinal motility in describing some digestive diseases.

Under normal circumstances, motility of the intestinal tract is different when food is present and when it is not present. When food is present, the small intestine engages in propulsion, moving food along from stomach to colon. Segmentation results when small areas of the intestine form a series of expanded areas and very narrow areas, forming what appear to be sausage links. Segmentation allows for mixing and breaking up material but does not actually push the ingesta very far along the tract. When food is not present, there is some very slow wave motion, most likely designed to get rid of any amounts of undigested material.

Transit time refers to the speed and nature of the motility of the intestines. If transit time is too fast, material will not have a chance to be digested and will come out as more liquid than solid. This is the case in diseases that cause diarrhea. If transit time is slow, material can come to obstruct the intestine. If transit time is slow through the colon in particular, the animal will be constipated.

The major function of the colon, in addition to funneling the material out of the body, is to resorb water. This is the body's last chance to reserve fluid before it is expelled from the body. When faced with the continuing presence of material in the distal colon, it will continue to withdraw more and more fluid. This is why feces from a constipated animal are small and hard; the water content has been almost totally removed. Unfortunately, the drier the feces, the harder it is to expel them, and the more time there is for water to be withdrawn. This condition is called constipation. This condition is treated with drugs called laxatives. Most laxatives have a high water content to rehydrate the fecal material; they also are thick, helping to draw the material along out of the body.

Recall that the anal sphincter has both smooth muscle and striated muscle sections. What this means is that the animal does have some voluntary control over defecation. By the same token, though, if the pressure to defecate is strong enough, it will overcome that control, and the smooth muscle section will open enough to cause feces to emerge. Inflammatory conditions put the control of these muscles under great stress. It is also of great importance if any surgery is done in the area of the anus. Interruption of the nerve controlling the anal sphincter can cause incontinence.

The liver

The liver is a highly vascularized organ that is involved in the majority of the bodily systems, including the digestive tract. The gallbladder produces bile, which is conducted through the liver by way of a series of small ducts until it reaches the duodenum.

The liver also participates directly in digestion in its role in filtering out material that has been resorbed from the intestines.

The enterohepatic circulation is also known as portal circulation. Some dogs are born with an abnormality in the vessels of the liver that affect the portal circulation. Instead of blood and waste products flowing back from the liver to the intestines, the material escapes through an abnormal blood vessel that shunts (diverts) the unwanted material into the systemic circulation. Known as a portosystemic shunt, it is characteristically associated with what appear to be neurological signs. This is because among the liver's roles is that of assisting with the breakdown of proteins. One of these breakdown products, ammonia, can be transported directly to the brain when a shunt of this type is present. Ammonia causes damage to the brain tissue and neurological signs emerge. The condition is surgically remediable.

Another role of the liver is the storage of glycogen. In times of stress, the liver can use this to assist in regulating blood glucose. A condition called diabetic ketoacidosis occurs when prolonged states of very low blood glucose occur. (This happens in a diabetic animal when insulin is not regulated well and/or given properly.) The liver will engage in the production of glucose to replenish the body's supply, in a process called gluconeogenesis. Unfortunately, if this continues over a long period of time, the liver can start to produce a by-product of this process known as a ketone. Ketones are damaging to any tissues that surround them, and also cause the pH of the blood to drop.

As alluded to earlier, the liver plays a role in filtering toxins. It also is able to break down many medications. This can make them easier for the body to use, or to eliminate. The liver also participates in the production of some of the elements that allow blood to clot. All of this is in addition to its role in assembling materials that are used to form feces.

In the dog, heart disease can affect the liver directly. This is because enlargement or inefficiency of the heart can cause a pressure "backup" in the vena cava, which passes near the liver on its way to the heart. This, in turn, causes pressure within the liver to increase dramatically. Fluid from within the soft tissue of the liver can actually be forced out of the liver and into the surrounding space of the abdomen. Ascites (fluid in the abdomen) can thus be caused by effusion of fluid from the liver, in response to cardiac disease.

Species differentiation

There are a few issues regarding other species that provide contrast to the system in dogs and cats. For example, equines and lagomorphs do most of their digestion in the cecum. The cecum (called the appendix in humans) has no function in dogs and cats. In horses and rabbits, however, the stomach actually does very little in terms of digestion. The cecum is relatively large in comparison to the cecum of dogs and cats, and it is crucial to their ability to metabolize food. Animals that are cecal digesters actually ferment their food rather than utilize the enzymes we discussed earlier. By the way, one of the reasons that horses and rabbits do not vomit is that the digested food is so far along in the system that it cannot work its way back to the surface.

The reader will have noticed that horses and rabbits have much in common from a metabolic standpoint.

The ruminant digestive system, as the reader will recall, has a four-chambered stomach, not four stomachs. It does not help that mammals like dogs and cats are referred to as monogastrics, implying that other species have more stomachs. The construction of the ruminant GI tract is designed to accommodate its diet in an extraordinary manner.

The cow subsists on a diet consisting mainly of cellulose (the major constituent of grass/hay). Cellulose (like fats) is hard to digest. From the outset, the bovine uses aggressive methods to break down food. The amount of amylase in cow saliva is multiplied many times compared to that in dogs. As amylase is designed to digest starch, it is clear that some aspects of digestion occur before the food reaches the stomach.

Material travels through the esophagus into the cranial-most part of the bovine stomach, known as the reticulum. It has a spongy appearance (humans do eat reticulum in some cultures, where it is known as tripe). The reticulum is positioned near the heart. The reticulum and the next chamber, the rumen, work together to process food. The rumen is the largest of the chambers. Food processed in these areas is returned to the oral cavity to be broken down further. A cow "chewing her cud" is regrinding her food and adding more amylase so that the pieces are small enough to be processed further.

The reticulum, rumen, and third chamber (omasum) are known as the forestomach. They contain a normal population of bacteria and fungi that help the enzymes present to process the cellulose. The cellulose is broken down to various saccharides, which, in turn, are used for energy.

The purpose of the forestomach is to process food by way of fermentation. This means that the process is anaerobic. In fact, the use of bacteria and fungus to break down sugars to carbon dioxide and fatty acids provides the main source of energy for the animal. (Proteins and other materials can also be utilized, but they form a small part of the diet.)

Fermentation is the main method of breaking down food in ruminants, equines, and lagomorphs. There is a "true stomach" in the ruminant, called the abomasum. This is a small section of the four-chambered stomach that performs some enzymatic functions similar to those of the dog and cat.

The pH balance in large animals is a more complex subject than in dogs and cats. Suffice it to say that rumen acidosis is a major problem in cattle, leading to illness and even death. In equines, it is believed that nutrition-related acidosis is a factor in laminitis, a hoof problem that is one of the leading reasons horses are euthanized due to the severity of its symptoms.

Clinical case resolution: Tarry stool

The dog mentioned earlier is producing feces with digested blood in it. It is this digested, dry blood that gives the stool its dark, sticky appearance. This type of fecal abnormality is called melena. Melena is not a disease; it merely refers to a description of the material. Its importance to us is that if the material has been at least partially digested, the problem resides in the stomach or the small intestine, not the colon. In this case, the dog had ingested a foreign body that caused ulceration in the stomach. The removal of the foreign body solved the problem.

Review questions

1 List three functions of the oral cavity not associated with digestion.
2 What is the purpose of the rugae?
3 Where does bile enter the intestinal tract? What does bile do?
4 What is the main digestive activity that occurs in the colon?
5 Does pH rise or fall as a dog or cat is digesting?
6 What is the name of the "true stomach" in the bovine?

Chapter 22 Endocrine Physiology

Clinical case: 9-year-old female dog

A 9-year-old female dog is brought into the clinic. Her family reports that she has been drinking a tremendous amount of water, and her urine volume has increased. She seems to be panting more often than usual. She has two symmetrical areas of alopecia along her back, and her abdomen seems to be distended when she is in a standing position.

Introduction

The various systems that control the metabolism of the animal are as intricate as they are interdependent. Careful study of even one system can be exhausting, and there are literally volumes written on each. In particular, the endocrine and neurological systems are so intertwined in their function that they are often referred to as a single unit, the "neuroendocrine" system. In the interest of making the material manageable, we will consider the endocrine system as a unit here. Bear in mind, however, that the functions of the endocrine and neurological systems are very closely related.

Endocrine glands

The endocrine glands are distinguished from other glands in the body in that they are ductless. The endocrine glands usually deliver their products directly into the bloodstream. The products of endocrine function are called hormones. They have the ability to initiate or catalyze reactions involving changes in metabolic rate, the autonomic nervous system, and the limbic system. There are discrete endocrine glands, organs that contain hormone-producing clusters of cells, or organs that have only patches of endocrine cells within them. Disorders of the endocrine system are among those most commonly encountered in small animal practice; these include over- or underproduction of hormones by the thyroid and adrenal glands, and manufacture of insufficient or poor quality insulin by the pancreas.

Hormones can be carried rapidly throughout the system and are able to cause significant change even in very small amounts. Certain cells in the body have a specific receptor (docking port)

Anatomy and Physiology for Veterinary Technicians and Nurses: A Clinical Approach, First Edition. Robin Sturtz and Lori Asprea.
© 2012 John Wiley & Sons, Inc. Published 2012 by John Wiley & Sons, Inc.

for a given hormone. The more receptors a cell has, the more sensitive it is to that hormone. By the same token, cells that do not have a receptor for, say, estrogen, will not be affected by it. Receptor cells for a given hormone may be grouped in one location or spread all over the body.

The receptors can actually change in their sensitivity to a hormone. The nervous system can upregulate (increase) or downregulate (decrease) the number of receptors that respond to a given hormone. This is part of the feedback loop that keeps the body from responding too much, or from failing to respond, to a given hormonal stimulus.

The pituitary

A discussion of the endocrine system should begin with the pituitary gland. While many of its functions are ultimately mediated by the hypothalamus, a center within the brain, it is the pituitary that is considered the endocrine "master gland." The pituitary sits ventral to the brain in a shallow depression of the braincase referred to as the sella turcica (for its supposed resemblance to a Turkish saddle).

The pituitary has a connection to the hypothalamus through a thin "stalk." The hypothalamus sits within the brain just rostral to the brain stem. The hypothalamus collects neural messages sent to the brain and funnels them in an organized manner to the pituitary gland. The releasing or inhibiting hormones it sends cause the pituitary to produce the appropriate hormones that go out to systemic endocrine organs via the bloodstream. The pituitary gland stimulates production, or directly produces, hormones associated with function of the heart, kidney, arterioles, adrenal glands, and reproductive system.

The pituitary (also known as the hypophysis) is divided into two functional sections: the anterior and posterior. If the hypothalamus sends a message to produce the hormones oxytocin and vasopressin, there will be stimulation of nerve endings within the posterior pituitary that will prompt the release of the required hormone.

The anterior pituitary produces a number of stimulating hormones. Thyroid-stimulating hormone (TSH) is the messenger sent to the thyroid gland to increase its activity. Adrenocorticotropic hormone (ACTH) stimulates function in the adrenal gland, where steroids and reproductive hormones are produced. The anterior pituitary also produces somatotropin (the root word soma referring to the body), also known as growth hormone (GH). Further, follicle-stimulating hormone (FSH), which is involved in the reproductive system, is sent out from the anterior pituitary (Box 22.1).

Box 22.1   Hormones and milk

At one time, synthetic GH was freely given to cows to increase milk production. Rising concern has curtailed this practice to some extent. The same GH that increases activity in the cow can also affect humans, but not always in a positive fashion. For example, excess GH can interfere with the cells' use of glucose and can cause hyperglycemia.

The posterior pituitary produces oxytocin, a hormone associated with parturition (giving birth) and "milk letdown" (when the mother's mammary glands start the process of getting milk from the mother to the infant).

Recall the discussion of vasopressin in surveying renal function. Vasopressin is a hormone. Vasopressin (also known as antidiuretic hormone [ADH]) has a direct effect on resorption of water within the kidney. In response to dehydration (increased osmotic pressure), the hormone is released and travels through the bloodstream, eventually reaching the kidneys. Specifically, it acts on the distal tubules of the nephron, with a particular effect on the water permeability of the collecting ducts. Aldosterone performs a similar function in that it causes sodium to be resorbed. As is usually the case, water will follow sodium out of cells and organs. Thus, the water is taken from the collecting duct before it is eliminated as urine and is brought back into the body where it can be used.

Another consequence of this function is that vasopressin helps maintain blood volume and thus systemic blood pressure. As more water is pulled back into the body from the nephron, it is added to the bloodstream. The increase in blood volume causes the heart contraction to increase in strength, increasing systemic blood pressure.

Vasopressin also affects systemic blood pressure by way of the size of the lumen of the veins. Vasopressin causes the veins to become smaller in diameter. The same amount of blood trying to get through a narrower vessel will naturally build up a great deal of pressure. Some medications meant to lower blood pressure are based on opposing this activity by relaxing the walls of the veins and/or by causing the kidney to release more water as a way of decreasing blood volume. These latter drugs, called diuretics, are commonly used in clinical practice.

Oxytocin has a number of functions, but its best-known purpose is to contribute to birth and lactation. Chapter 24 will go into greater depth on this subject. For the moment, though, we can point out that at a certain point toward the end of pregnancy, oxytocin is released from the pituitary in fairly large amounts. This causes contraction of the walls of the uterus in mammals and thus assists in the process of birth. As mentioned earlier, it also causes contractions within the mammary gland/udder that allow milk to be accessed by the newborn.

The thyroid

The thyroid gland produces two major hormones. One, thyroid hormone, has a wide range of activities that together control much of the body's metabolic rate. The other, calcitonin, is a more specific hormone that has to do with calcium levels in the body.

Calcitonin is produced in the C cells of the thyroid. When excessive levels of calcium are sensed in the bloodstream, the hormone is released. It will act to deposit calcium within bone throughout the body. Along with the parathyroid gland, it has a strong influence on the balance of calcium and phosphorus in the body. Given the importance of calcium for cell metabolism and neuronal function, this is no small task.

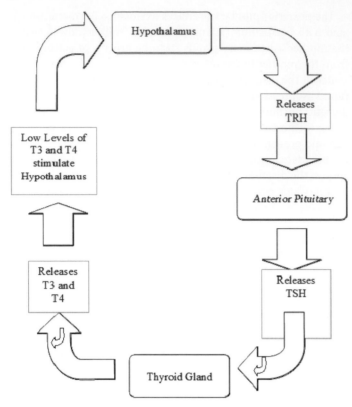

Figure 22.1   The hypothalamic-pituitary-thyroid loop. As T3 and T4 levels drop, the hypothalamus will signal for increased output. If levels of T3/T4 rise excessively, as in hyperthyroidism, the hypothalamus will stop sending TRH so as to step down thyroid hormone production.

The thyroid gland contains groups of cells called follicles. They help produce thyroglobulin, which is the base from which the hormones thyroxin (T4) and triiodothyronine (T3) are manufactured. This process starts with the hypothalamus producing a hormone called thyroid-releasing hormone (TRH). This, in turn, signals the pituitary to produce TSH, which is released to the thyroid gland to cause it to produce T4 and T3. See Figure 22.1 for a diagram of the feedback loop involved.

This process is not possible without the presence of iodide. In fact, the mammalian body needs iodides as part of its diet. The fact that any iodine that enters the system is taken up by the thyroid is the basis for the treatment of hyperthyroidism. In order to treat hyperthyroidism so that the client does not have to administer medication at home, radioactive iodine is administered; it goes directly to the thyroid and ablates the overactive parts of the gland, eliminating the need for medication to control the overproduction of the hormones.

The presence of feedback loops is an important part of the function of the endocrine system. The thyroid provides a good example of this. TSH is sent to the thyroid, which causes it to produce T3 and T4. Much of the T4 is converted to T3 during metabolism. When blood levels of T3 rise to a certain point, this will be noticed by the pituitary gland. The pituitary then

suppresses the production of TSH, which, in turn, ensures that less thyroid hormone is sent out into the system. In short, the pituitary tells the thyroid to secrete hormone, which causes metabolic rates to rise. When T3 levels rise high enough, the pituitary takes this as a sign to stop sending a stimulating message to the thyroid. This kind of balance is referred to as a negative feedback loop, meaning that at a certain point, information from the body is fed back to the central nervous system and the central nervous system suppresses whatever function is in high gear.

Most thyroid hormone is circulating in the bloodstream bound to proteins. A very small amount of T4 (and even less T3) is unbound or "free" within the blood. It is the free form that actually enters the cells to regulate metabolic rate at a cellular level. When more hormone is needed by the cells, the hormone is released from the blood proteins so that it is available for uptake. In fact, the level of free T4 is one measure the pituitary uses to direct the feedback loop. We take advantage of this system when we test animals for hyperthyroidism and hypothyroidism. The amount of T4 circulating in the bloodstream is a good indicator of thyroid function. Measurement of free T4 is even more specific.

A normal thyroid gland releases mostly the T4 form into the bloodstream. The T4 molecule is converted to T3 by a change in the iodide content of the molecule. Certain changes will create a T3 that upregulates (increases) the level of cellular activity. Other changes lead to a type of T3 that decreases the activity in a cell. Thus, the thyroid is very much like the accelerator of a car; it can speed up or slow down the production of energy in cells in the kidney, heart, and so on, to increase or decrease their activity.

While the thyroid gland affects almost every body system, it has a particular effect on the following:

Heart: rate and rhythm
Respiration: rate and efficiency
Digestion: rate
Growth: fetal development

The thyroid hormone influences the concentration and activity of many enzymes as well. Directly or indirectly, it affects the basic activity level of all major systems.

The phenomenon of "sick euthyroid" laboratory findings is a reflection of the complexity of these relationships. Under ordinary circumstances, a healthy animal produces a certain amount of thyroid hormone. In an animal with chronic illness, however, thyroid hormone levels may be low without any thyroid disease. The condition is not clearly understood; theories include decreased release of TSH or failure of the T4 and/or T3 to bind to proteins in the blood in a normal manner.

The parathyroid

The parathyroid glands sit on or within the thyroid gland. Their main function is to produce parathormone (PTH). PTH is basically the opposite of calcitonin. PTH works to counteract hypocalcemia by taking calcium out of the bones (and helping to resorb it from the kidneys), putting more of it into circulation.

Many lizards have a need for a high level of calcium in their diet. If they do not get enough calcium, they will overproduce PTH in an effort to bring more calcium into the bloodstream so it can be used by the cells for energy. This weakens the bones considerably.

The adrenal gland

The adrenal gland plays a major role in three specific areas: the autonomic nervous system, the reproductive system, and general metabolic rate and efficiency. The adrenal gland responds to the hormone ACTH, released from the anterior pituitary gland. Its cortex (superficial layers) has three zones, which produce several types of hormones: glucocorticoids, mineralocorticoids, and sex hormones (androgens and estrogens) (Figure 10.3). All of these have a common chemical structure and fall into the category of steroids. Note that steroid hormones are manufactured in part with the use of cholesterol. While too much cholesterol is undesirable, too little is also a problem.

The adrenal medulla releases the hormones epinephrine and norepinephrine (or adrenalin and noradrenalin; the names are interchangeable). Epinephrine is the basis for the sympathetic nervous system response to the environment. Anything that is exciting or threatening to the animal will trigger certain pathways within the central nervous system that instruct the adrenal gland to release epinephrine. The hormone is a strong stimulant and increases the activity of the heart, respiratory tract, and muscular systems. In its capacity as a neurotransmitter, it also puts the rest of the body on alert for sudden changes. Refer to Chapter 18 for the relative functions of the sympathetic and parasympathetic nervous systems.

The glucocorticoids are important because they stimulate functions like gluconeogenesis, which refers to the process of manufacturing glucose. They also have strong anti-inflammatory properties. As inflammation is caused by the immune system, in response to a disease or injury, what glucocorticoids do in effect is suppress the immune system. The glucocorticoids include cortisol and corticosterone. As suggested earlier, many drugs are based on the action of these molecules and their properties.

On the other hand, glucocorticoids inhibit the formation of fibroblasts, which are important in wound healing. An animal receiving therapeutic glucocorticoid drugs or who has a hyperactive adrenal gland will not heal as quickly or completely as a healthy animal. This is an important issue in wound management in the clinic.

Glucocorticoids are also indirectly involved in the "stress response." They can be associated with an increase in systemic blood pressure.

One of the most common metabolic diseases in dogs is hyperadrenocorticism (Cushing's disease). Either because of abnormality in the adrenal gland or the pituitary gland, the output of many adrenal hormones increases dramatically. Patients can present with weight loss, skin and haircoat changes, vomiting and diarrhea, and an increase in drinking and urinating. This last phenomenon is known as PUPD, short for polyuria (urinating large amounts) and polydipsia (drinking large amounts). While PUPD is associated with dozens of diseases, it is a classic symptom of hyperadrenocorticism. Cushing's disease is seen in horses and cats, but nowhere near as commonly as in dogs.

Pituitary-dependent Cushing's disease is a condition whereby there is dysfunction of the pituitary, causing it to send out excessive ACTH. Usually, this dysfunction is related to the presence of a benign tumor, although there are rare instances of malignancy. The high levels of ACTH cause the adrenal gland to produce high levels of steroid hormones. These hormones cause increased levels of protein and glucose in the blood, the former the result of catabolism (breaking down existing proteins) and the latter because of the push to gluconeogenesis (producing glucose). The glucocorticoids, in particular, also suppress the immune system. The combination of these changes is what leads to the clinical signs.

The difficulty lies in the fact that the high levels of steroid hormone production cause the adrenal gland to increase in size, a phenomenon called hyperplasia. The bigger the gland, the more hormones it puts out, exacerbating the problem. Note that there can be hyperplasia of the adrenal gland in the absence of any problem with the pituitary. In fact, this is quite common.

Under ordinary circumstances, the high levels of steroid would trigger the hypothalamus to order the pituitary gland to stop sending out ACTH. Unfortunately, at a high enough steroid level, the pituitary (and perhaps even the hypothalamus) is not able to respond, and the feedback loop ceases to be effective.

In fact, one of the ways we test for the presence of Cushing's disease is to administer a steroid called dexamethasone. Its presence in the bloodstream should cause the pituitary to stop pumping out ACTH. Therefore, the blood level of steroid hormones in the system should drop over the next few hours. If no such drop occurs, the feedback loop is not working. In essence, steroid hormones are at such high levels that administering more has no effect.

The disease resulting from insufficient adrenal gland function is Addison's disease, or hypoadrenocorticism. This too is most common in dogs but is seen in cats as well. It is associated with weight gain and a low activity level. It is more common for the issue to be the decrease in adrenal function, but there can be an insufficiency in the pituitary as well.

Causes of adrenal gland atrophy may include immune-mediated disease or may be the result of an unknown mechanism. Perhaps the most common cause, though, is iatrogenic. In giving steroid medications, treating anything from allergy to cancer, we sometimes cause the adrenal gland to stop functioning. Basically, the high level of steroid in the blood occasioned by the drug causes the pituitary to stop producing ACTH, which stops stimulation to the adrenal. Without stimulation, the organ can atrophy, just like a muscle would if it were not used. As a result, when the gland is needed, it may not respond. The animal gains weight, is slow-moving, and appears depressed. He is unable to mount a strong response to environmental stimulation, as he cannot increase his supply of glucose.

The most important mineralocorticoid is aldosterone. It plays a key role in prompting the kidney to resorb sodium, once again allowing the body to conserve water. It also promotes the excretion of ions like potassium and hydrogen. Hydrogen balance is important in maintaining pH (the relatively acid or alkaline nature of the blood). Potassium is particularly important in the transmission of nerve impulses and in muscle function. As we have noted, keeping potassium levels in check is a key element of healthy metabolism. Excess potassium can be fatal. In fact, it is a component of many euthanasia solutions.

In cases of hypoadrenocorticism, aldosterone production is also compromised. This impairs the kidney's ability to reserve sodium and to excrete potassium, as those functions are mediated by aldosterone. There is a condition called Addisonian crisis that results from this electrolyte imbalance. The dog will exhibit signs of weakness, bradycardia (slow heart rate), hypoglycemia (low blood glucose level), and possibly even seizures. It is referred to as a crisis because, if left untreated, even for a short time, it can result in the death of the patient.

Recall that aldosterone is part of the renin–angiotensin–aldosterone (RAA) system. When the kidney senses low blood pressure, it will release renin, which is made in cells near the glomerulus. Renin, in turn, leads to the production of angiotensin. Among the other steps that this triggers is the production of aldosterone. By acting on the kidney to keep fluid content within the body, aldosterone helps increase blood volume and thus blood pressure.

One of the steps in the production of angiotensin involves the participation of an enzyme called angiotensin-converting enzyme (ACE). The purpose of the RAA system is to raise blood pressure. Thus, a drug that could counteract ACE would interrupt the RAA system and help reduce blood pressure. Drugs like this are called ACE inhibitors and are widely used in cases of hypertension. Interestingly, the first ACE inhibitor was developed as a result of studies of the Brazilian pit viper, a snake that kills by causing a catastrophic drop in blood pressure. Its method of doing this was a natural form of an ACE-inhibiting molecule.

The adrenal medulla produces epinephrine and norepinephrine. When the sympathetic nervous system is called into play, the adrenal gland releases these hormones. They cause all of the activities we associate with the sympathetic part of the autonomic nervous system: increased heart rate and blood pressure, widened bronchi, and decreased digestive activity.

As indicated at the beginning of this chapter, there can be endocrine tissue within other organs, as opposed to the whole organ being dedicated just to hormone production. A good example of this is the pancreas.

The pancreas and insulin

The part of the pancreas that produces digestive enzymes is known as the exocrine pancreas. This distinguishes it from the endocrine pancreas, the parts of the pancreas that produce hormones. The endocrine pancreas produces insulin, glucagon, and somatostatin. The latter inhibits the production of insulin. Insulin and glucagon have to do with the use of glucose.

The B cells, which are within areas of the pancreas called the islets of Langerhans, produce insulin. The production of insulin is triggered by high levels of glucose or amino acids in the blood, digestive activity, and/or parasympathetic nerve stimulation.

Insulin serves to escort the glucose within the bloodstream into the cells of the body so that the glucose can be used to create energy. When insulin levels are insufficient, or when the insulin is of poor quality, or if the cells of the body become resistant to it, excess glucose remains in the bloodstream. High levels of glucose in the bloodstream, so high that the glucose spills out in the urine, is the disease state known as diabetes mellitus. (As an aside, it is important to use both words here. There is another kind of diabetes, called diabetes insipidus, which has nothing to do with the pancreas.)

Glucagon production, on the other hand, is stimulated by the condition of low levels of glucose in the bloodstream or by the sympathetic nervous system. When glucagon is released by the pancreas and reaches the liver, it stimulates the liver to break down the compound glycogen, which results in the production of more glucose.

Other endocrine activities

There are also hormone-producing cells in the kidney. Erythropoietin is a hormone that is produced in response to a low level of red blood cells in the bloodstream. This hormone stimulates the bone marrow to produce more red blood cells. It is not surprising, then, that animals with chronic renal disease often become anemic. The malfunctioning kidney does not make erythropoietin in sufficient quantities, or perhaps does not make it at all, and the animal has an insufficient supply of oxygen-carrying cells.

Pheromones are hormones in the sense that they are chemical messengers that stimulate reactions, but they work outside rather than inside the body in terms of their effect. Pheromones are only detected by members of the same species as the one producing them. Felines are able to distinguish feline pheromones, but humans are not sensitive to them. Pheromones are associated with a wide range of behaviors, some related to the reproductive cycle and some to emotional state. Certain pheromones have a calming effect, for example.

Clinical case resolution: 9-year-old female dog

The case cited at the beginning is, in fact, a case of hyperadreno-corticism or Cushing's disease. It is particularly common in older dogs and is associated with weight loss, a distended abdomen (loss of skin turgor), and symmetrical alopecia (hair loss). Seeing these signs should alert the clinician to consider adrenal and/or pituitary disease as a possible cause of the problem..

Review questions

1 When calcitonin is active, would you expect blood levels of calcium to rise or fall?
2 What does oxytocin do? What particular type of muscle does it affect?
3 What is a negative feedback loop?
4 Would the administration of steroid-based drugs interfere with wound healing? Why?
5 What are the islets of Langerhans?
6 What would happen if the cells of the body were resistant to insulin?
7 Where is epinephrine produced?
8 Do endocrine glands have ducts? If not, how do hormones get to their targets?
9 What does glucagon do?

Chapter 23 Respiratory Physiology

Clinical case: Dog in respiratory distress

A dog is brought into the clinic in respiratory distress. He is panting, slow-moving, and stands in an orthopneic position. These symptoms are a demonstration of what goes wrong when normal functions are disrupted.

Introduction

Respiratory systems have at their core a basic definition. In order to pull air into the animal so that oxygen can be extracted and spread to the tissues, a series of chemical and mechanical steps are necessary. By the same token, a pathway for expelling carbon dioxide must be available. Other materials such as water vapor are also inhaled and exhaled.

The basics

A few definitions are in order. Ventilation refers to the movement of air/gases into and out of the respiratory tract. It is not a specific quantitative measure but a description of a general action.

Tidal volume actually refers to measurement. Tidal volume is the amount of air that is moved with each breath. Minute ventilation is an even more specific number; it is the total amount of air that is breathed in and out in 1 minute. Minute volume is calculated by multiplying tidal volume by breaths per minute (BPM). In effect, if either the total amount of air being moved or the rate at which it is moving varies, minute ventilation will be affected. The clinical significance of this lies in disease states or medication effects that change the depth or shallowness of breathing, and/or change the respiration rate (BPM). For example, hyperthermia (fever) will often cause panting, as the

Anatomy and Physiology for Veterinary Technicians and Nurses: A Clinical Approach, First Edition. Robin Sturtz and Lori Asprea.
© 2012 John Wiley & Sons, Inc. Published 2012 by John Wiley & Sons, Inc.

body attempts to decrease its core temperature. As a result, the minute ventilation will be adversely affected in that abnormally rapid rates of air intake do not allow for large amounts to be inhaled.

Another important term is "dead space." Dead space refers to areas of the respiratory tract in which there is no active gas exchange. There are two kinds: anatomical and physiological.

The term "anatomical dead space" refers to the area from the entrance to the respiratory system at the nares through the major bronchi. This area serves to conduct air into the lungs. It does not move oxygen or other gases on a cellular level, as is the case in the alveoli of the lungs. While respiration is dependent upon the channeling of air to the alveoli, the space is considered dead in that there is no exchange of oxygen and carbon dioxide at this level. Were it not for the anatomical dead space, air would have to be conducted to the lungs through the skin (as is the case in some amphibians) or by some artificial means such as a tracheostomy tube.

Physiological dead space is related to the alveoli themselves, where the actual exchange of gases occurs. Not all alveoli are perfused to the same degree; that is, some of them are inactive at any given time, and there is no gas exchange taking place. If only as a result of the effects of gravity and movement, the capillary blood supply to each alveolus is different. The ones that are not perfused sufficiently (do not have much blood passing by) do not actively engage in gas exchange.

The combination of anatomical dead space and alveolar dead space is referred to as physiological dead space. The more physiological dead space, the less surface area there is for the animal to exchange carbon dioxide and oxygen to a sufficient degree for normal function. A particular concern arises during surgery, when the animal is intubated. The endotracheal (breathing) tube itself is dead space. Using a tube that is too long or too wide interferes with the motion needed for respiration and may provoke decreased gas exchange, even though the animal is receiving oxygen directly into the airway. It is for this reason (among others) that we monitor oxygen and carbon dioxide levels in the blood during surgery.

One other point needs to be made in reference to ventilation. Once gases reach the alveoli, they are processed so that some elements are absorbed into the bloodstream and others passed into the alveolus so that they can be exhaled. This exchange, as noted above, happens by way of local blood vessels. If the minute ventilation of the animal is too high or too low relative to the rate and amount of blood flowing past the alveolus, the gas exchange will be inefficient. Put another way, if the amount of air exchanged does not match the ability of blood to pick up oxygen and discharge carbon dioxide, the "hand-off" of gases does not go smoothly. This is referred to as ventilation/perfusion (V/Q) mismatch. A slight amount of mismatch is normal in a healthy animal, as BPM and rate of blood flow are variable enough in the normal animal that they do not match up at all times. However, an abnormal amount of V/Q mismatch makes it harder to get oxygen into the body.

Ventilation and temperature

A major factor in the changeable nature of minute ventilation is the interplay of ambient (outside the body) and core temperature. An animal suffering from heat stress, as the febrile animal we discussed earlier, will decrease activity in an effort to avoid building up more heat. This result is obtained because decreasing activity increases the amount of dead space, which allows the animal to shed heat. In contrast, a hypothermic animal will evidence a slower respiratory rate but an increase in tidal volume. This increases the efficiency of the gas exchange and allows the animal to increase metabolic energy production—in short, to warm up.

Considering the animal under anesthesia again, it should now be evident that another corollary of increasing dead space is that the animal will shed heat. An animal under anesthesia is already experiencing a decrease in core temperature as metabolic activity is slowed by the drug. Add to that more heat loss through an inappropriately placed endotracheal tube, and the problem of surgical hypothermia will be even worse. Warming blankets or other devices are often used during or after surgery to counteract this problem.

Residual capacity

Functional residual capacity is a phrase that refers to the fact that there is a small amount of air that remains in the lungs after exhalation. This amount of air helps maintain the slightly negative air pressure in the chest cavity, relative to air pressure outside the body. The consistency of the level of air in the cavity is enough to ensure that ventilation will be relatively consistent with the animal at rest. As is true for all body systems, regular rhythms contribute to consistency (see Figure 23.1).

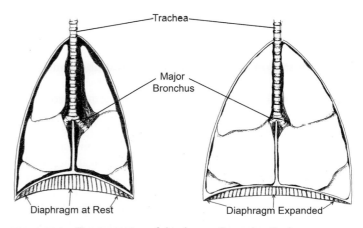

Figure 23.1   The expansion of the thorax allows the diaphragm to expand, and the pressure change brings air into the lungs. Exhalation in dogs and cats is passive, and so the diaphragm returns to its resting position without external force.

Thoracic pressure

If the chest cavity is punctured, say, by traumatic injury, the balance between the air pressure inside and outside of the body is now changed as more air enters the cavity. This increased pressure will cause the lung to collapse down in size. The collapse of a lung is called atelectasis. It is actually more likely in thoracic injury to a young animal than an older animal. Adult tissue is stiffer and less likely to collapse. There are other causes of atelectasis, but this one is germane to our discussion.

As the thoracic cavity expands and contracts during mammalian respiration, the diaphragm moves. The muscles of inhalation include the external intercostals and the scalenus muscle. The diaphragm is active during inhalation and recoils (passively returns) during exhalation. It is a musculotendinous tissue, having both strength and flexibility. As muscles contract to allow the animal to inhale, the diaphragm is drawn caudally and flattens. This helps increase the size of the thoracic cavity. The expansion causes the relative air pressure in the thorax to be even lower than that of the ambient air. The condition of negative air pressure in the thorax is an enticement for air from the outside to come in.

Once the muscles have reached their furthest expansion, they will stop. The elastic properties of the lungs and the thoracic cavity will cause these tissues to rebound to their normal position. The diaphragm will also recoil to its relaxed position and take on a curved appearance. This will cause air to be expelled from the animal.

The process of exhalation in dogs and cats is, for the most part, passive. It is not so much the force of muscle contracting as it is the return to a resting state that causes air to flow out of the respiratory system. There is some minor contribution, however, to exhalation by muscles such as the internal intercostals.

The nervous system and respiration

In an animal that is having difficulty breathing, the central nervous system will attempt to apply more muscular force to inhalation. For example, additional abdominal muscles will be recruited. Large excursions of the chest and abdomen denote increased respiratory effort and are a clear marker for respiratory disease/distress in a patient who presents with this symptom.

Another factor assisting the movement of the lungs during respiration is the presence of a scant amount of viscous fluid between the parietal and visceral pleura. This provides lubrication for the movement of the tissues.

There is another relevant point regarding the movement of air through the respiratory apparatus. As the flow of air approaches the alveoli, it is going through narrower airways. This causes airflow to slow down considerably and make less noise as it is moving. As a result, when auscultating the thorax in the normal animal, what is being heard (in terms of respiratory sounds) is mostly the upper respiratory tract (to the level of the major bronchi) rather than the bronchioles. This is why thoracic radiographs are so important in diagnosing respiratory disease. While auscultation may not yield anything remarkable, clear abnormalities may be identified on diagnostic imaging.

The rhythmicity of breathing

The rate and volume of air inhaled and exhaled during respiration is mediated by many factors, some of which have already been noted. There are other features that also participate.

Within the lung parenchyma (the specific cells associated with the organ and their supporting connective tissue), there are stretch receptors. These receptors are also present in the airways, and even the surrounding musculature. For example, as the lungs fill with air, the stretch receptors sense the expansion and signal the nervous system regarding the degree of movement.

Cilia are small hairs. There are ciliated cells in many parts of the body, including the respiratory system and the inner ear. In the case of the respiratory system, they are present in the trachea and in the major bronchi. These cells are very responsive to the touch of anything other than air, such as particulate matter that has been inhaled. When they are touched, they generate an action potential that signals the central nervous system to change respiratory rate and rhythm.

The autonomic nervous system plays a large role in the function of the respiratory system. There is smooth muscle from the trachea all the way down to the alveoli. The smooth muscle within the bronchi and bronchioles responds to parasympathetic stimulation from the vagus nerve (cranial nerve X). Acetylcholine is released, which causes the muscle to contract and thus constrict the airway. This, in turn, will cause changes in air intake, which may have been triggered by the central nervous system perceiving hypoxia. In contrast, there is also sympathetic innervation to the smooth muscle. Triggering these neurotransmitters will cause dilation of the airways.

Gas exchange

Just as the pressure within the chest leads to inhalation or exhalation, gas exchange itself is based on pressure differentials. Gas exchange includes a number of molecules. For our purposes, the term "gas exchange" refers to the delivery of oxygen to the bloodstream and the infiltration of carbon dioxide into the alveolus so that it can be exhaled (see Figure 23.2). We generally talk about partial pressure, which refers to the pressure of a particular gas relative to the overall gas/air pressure of the surrounding area. The abbreviation Pa is used to indicate partial pressure. Thus, PaO_2 is the partial pressure of oxygen in an area, and $PaCO_2$ is the partial pressure of carbon dioxide.

Note that neither PaO_2 nor $PaCO_2$ is a static number. PaO_2 will necessarily fluctuate with inhalation and exhalation. The amount of oxygen, and thus its pressure, will vary based on how much air is entering or leaving the system. In fact, the exchange of oxygen and carbon dioxide that occurs between the alveolus and the capillary is the source of fluctuation of oxygen pressure in the alveolus itself.

Despite the fluctuation, the alveolus will normally have a higher PaO_2 than the capillaries flowing past it. The blood

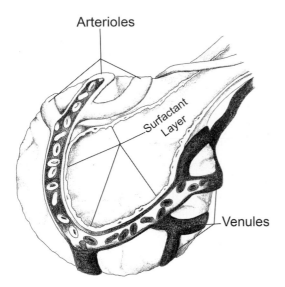

Figure 23.2   The alveolus. The venules and arterioles pass around the alveolus, and gases are exchanged across the surface of the interior.

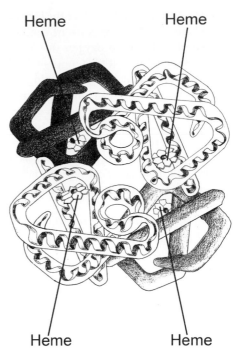

Figure 23.3   A molecule of hemoglobin has four heme units (or "hemes").

flowing from the heart to the lung is carrying a very low PaO_2, the oxygen having been depleted by the body as the blood passes through the animal. The oxygen will diffuse from where its pressure is the highest (the alveolus) to the capillaries, where PaO_2 is lower. The reverse occurs with $PaCO_2$, which is higher in the capillaries than in the alveoli.

One of the things that make the surface of the alveolus permeable to gases is a material on its luminal surface called surfactant. Puppies or kittens (or humans, for that matter) that are born prematurely have not developed a sufficient layer of surfactant and thus have significant neonatal respiratory distress.

Certain diseases and toxins can alter the permeability of the alveoli. In inflammatory conditions, the gas exchange is less efficient as a result of the increased thickness of the swollen tissues. One of the basic principles underlying the administration of pure oxygen to an animal with respiratory distress is the increase of PaO_2 that results within the alveolus. This strengthens the ability of the oxygen to cross the alveolar border and to enter the capillary. The increased movement of oxygen into the bloodstream will allow more CO_2 to diffuse out of the bloodstream.

Having discussed pressure ratios in a little more detail, it is time to return to the subject of the V/Q mismatch. If the normal function of the respiratory system depends on the gas pressure and the speed of the bloodstream being ideally synchronized, anything that interferes with that match may make gas transfer less efficient. Potential interferences with V/Q matching include increased cardiac output. It is akin to trying to catch a taxi while it is still moving by; the greater speed and volume of blood passing by the alveolus hinder the efficiency of the gas exchange.

The other side of this problem is that of insufficient BPM. If the PaO_2 is not high enough in the alveolus, it will not cross over to the capillaries. Animals who have been exercising will often pant; this increases oxygen intake by way of increasing respira-

tory rate, in an effort to balance out the increased cardiac output that accompanies exercise. Note that panting without sufficient tidal volume will create a significant deficit in the alveolar PaO_2.

Hemoglobin

Once the blood is oxygenated, it returns to the heart so that it can be pumped out into the body. However, oxygen is poorly soluble in water. Very little of it will enter the plasma, and thus it would be difficult for it to get into the cells of the body. The solution to this is a molecule called hemoglobin.

Hemoglobin is a pigmented molecule that has four substructures called hemes. Each heme is associated with a particular protein (see Figure 23.3). These proteins are the same within a given species of animal, but usually differ among species. The hemoglobin is a constituent of the red blood cell. Its pigment is what gives the cell its characteristic color; the oxidation of the iron within the pigment leads to the color change.

Since there are four hemes for each molecule of hemoglobin, and each heme holds a molecule of oxygen, each red blood cell carries four oxygen molecules. Multiplying the number of red blood cells (erythrocytes) by four will yield the amount of oxygen the bloodstream is carrying. Given that there are millions of red blood cells in a typical dog or cat, the number is impressive.

Another constituent of hemoglobin is iron molecules. Anemia (the condition of having insufficient red blood cells) can be associated with iron deficiency. Animals with severe anemia are often given iron supplements in recognition of this concept.

Hemoglobin acquires oxygen by way of the binding of oxygen to the heme, mediated by the ferrous (iron) components of the hemoglobin molecule. The more oxygen that is acquired, the more readily the hemoglobin will take more in. This phenomenon is called affinity. It is analogous to opening a door a little wider each time a person comes in until all four people have come in (i.e., all four hemes have attached to oxygen).

Thus, oxygen is carried through the bloodstream by hemoglobin. At some point, it needs to dissociate itself from the blood so that it can be taken up by the tissues. The oxyhemoglobin dissociation curve is a mathematical representation of what it takes for the oxygen molecules to "free themselves" from the hemoglobin.

Hemoglobin does have a limit to how much oxygen it can carry. When the hemoglobin is at 100% of its carrying capacity, it is said to be saturated. As the blood leaves the lungs, the hemoglobin is close to its saturation point. Traveling through the body, the oxygen will be drawn off whenever the surrounding tissue has a relatively low amount of oxygen (low oxygen pressure). This is known as the dissociation point.

The exact amount of oxygen that reaches the dissociation point is not a fixed number. Several factors have an effect on how many oxygen molecules have to build up before they "jump off" the hemoglobin. For one thing, the dissociation point varies depending on the relative oxygenation of the tissue that surrounds it. If the local cells are full of oxygen, there is not enough of a pressure difference to encourage the oxygen to leave the hemoglobin.

In anemia, the overall carrying capacity of oxygen in the blood is diminished. Because not much oxygen is getting to the tissues, it does not take much for there to be a big difference between the oxygen pressure in the hemoglobin and that in the tissues. Once there is enough of a difference, the oxygen will dissociate. Since the oxygen dissociates sooner than it ordinarily would (say, by the time it gets to the abdominal organs), the hemoglobin that gets around to the later parts of the system has already depleted its reserves.

When an animal is hyperthermic, the increased temperature of the blood will make it easier for oxygen to dissociate. The point at which the ratio of hemoglobin oxygen concentration, and body tissue oxygen concentration, will be more favorable occurs at a lower level of oxygen when there are higher local temperatures. In essence, it is easier to off-load the oxygen at a higher blood temperature.

The reverse is true when the animal is hypothermic. The oxygen pressure in the tissues of the body must be lower than normal in order for oxygen to dissociate from the hemoglobin. Warming the animal gradually will allow the normal gradient (relative amount of difference between one thing and another) of oxygen pressure to reassert itself so the dissociation point returns to normal.

Unfortunately, oxygen is not the only thing that binds to hemoglobin. Carbon monoxide has 200 times the binding capacity to heme that oxygen does. Animals exposed to high levels of carbon monoxide will have so much of it bound to their heme that there will be no room for oxygen to bind with it. Nitrites and other toxins can bind to the iron in the heme and also prevent the binding of oxygen to the hemoglobin. Nitrites are a particular problem in ruminant feeds in that they are found as a contaminant in food that has been poorly processed or stored.

Carbon dioxide

Just as the blood that enters systemic circulation from the left ventricle is heavily oxygenated, the blood that enters the venous system has dropped off most of its oxygen and is now carrying the metabolic by-product carbon dioxide. Carbon dioxide can be carried in solution in the blood. It can also be carried in the cytoplasm of the red blood cell in the form of its metabolites, bicarbonate and oxygen. In fact, when blood is analyzed chemically in standard clinical practice, the measurement of bicarbonate levels is used to infer levels of carbon dioxide in the blood. The measurement of carbon dioxide is much more difficult than the measure of bicarbonate.

As the venous blood circulates and arrives at the alveoli, the CO_2 pressure is much higher in the bloodstream than in the alveoli. It will thus be drawn into the alveolus, where the $PaCO_2$ is normally low.

Carbon dioxide can cause significant illness if not expelled from the body. High levels of carbon dioxide in the bloodstream result in acidemia, or low blood pH. Anything that impedes the exchange of gases across the alveolar boundary, such as pulmonary disease, can result in acidemia. Increased respiratory rate is a method of literally blowing out more carbon dioxide in an attempt to raise blood pH. The term respiratory acidosis refers to the increase in blood levels of carbon dioxide associated with the inability of the lung to absorb and eliminate this gas.

Respiratory alkalosis is associated with hyperventilation. In cases of hypoxia or pulmonary disease, respiratory rate will increase. In this case, carbon dioxide leaves the body at a greater than normal rate, and the body is not able to keep up with its production. Having less than a normal amount of carbon dioxide in the lung is actually problematic in that it raises blood pH. Some normal metabolic functions are only possible with pH at an optimal level. Therefore, either respiratory alkalosis or acidosis is a problem. Testing of blood pH is easily done with conventional blood testing equipment.

Chemoreceptors

The chemoreceptors are in various locations. They monitor the relative amounts of oxygen and carbon dioxide in the bloodstream, as well as blood pH. Chemoreceptors are located in the carotid and aortic bodies, and in the medulla oblongata.

The carotid body is a collection of receptors near the branching of the external and internal carotid arteries. The aortic body is, not surprisingly, seated in connective tissue around the aortic arch. They are particularly responsive to hypoxia (low levels of oxygen), hypercapnia (high levels of carbon dioxide), and acidemia (low pH). The central chemoreceptors are present on the ventrolateral surface of the medulla oblongata. This area is even more sensitive to carbon dioxide levels.

The carotid body is actually more active in juveniles, and the aortic body in older animals. The medulla of the brain is very sensitive to pH throughout the animal's life. Together, these chemoreceptors monitor blood gases and pH, and help determine respiratory rate and tidal volume. The information from these areas is also used by the renal system. When pH is sensed as being too high, the renal tubules will excrete more bicarbonate (which is alkaline).

Mechanisms to increase oxygenation

If a lack of oxygen is sensed by the chemoreceptors, there are a number of resources with which to work. As noted earlier, increasing core temperature will encourage oxygen dissociation from hemoglobin, making more of it available. Increasing cardiac output will also help. The increased amount of blood in circulation allows for the availability of more oxygen.

Two minor ways are also available for increasing oxygen supplies. One is splenic contraction. The spleen has a large number of erythrocytes in it, which, in turn, carry oxygen as they normally do. The organ can contract, and add to the total blood volume. This is only a minor contribution.

As noted in Chapter 16, one of the materials in skeletal muscle is something called myoglobin. Myoglobin does have a small store of oxygen in it. If the oxygen level of the blood brought to the muscle is not enough, the myoglobin can contribute at least a little so that muscle function may continue.

Species differences

Fish, amphibians, and lizards all have somewhat different respiratory systems, and all differ from those of mammals. Avians, however, are unique.

The body of the bird contains air sacs, extending from the neck to the caudal abdomen. It is the air sacs that do the contraction and expansion that draws air in and pushes it out of the body. While the actual gas exchange is done in the lung, just as in a mammal, the lung is relatively quite small and does not undergo any rhythmic change in size or shape (see Figure 23.4).

As the main bronchus travels cranially to caudally, it runs through the entire horizontal axis of the lung. It gives off airways of diminishing diameter, fed by the air sacs, which are eventually the size of capillaries. These air capillaries are paired with blood capillaries in the lung, and gas exchange occurs across their surfaces.

The air sacs are large enough, and the lung parenchyma is dense enough, that rupture of one area of the air sac is not enough to cause atelectasis. On the other hand, the tissue of the air sacs, which have the appearance of Bubble Wrap, is rather delicate. This fact, coupled with the necessity of strong muscle contraction so that the entire system of air sacs can move as one, has great clinical significance. When restraining a bird for examination, it is important not to hold the body of the bird too tightly, particularly in the mid-thorax. Excess pressure on the muscles of inhalation will strangle the bird as the lung has no way to draw air in for itself.

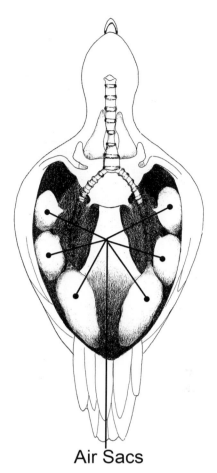

Air Sacs

Figure 23.4   The air sacs expand and contract, and allow for the flow of air. The lungs are interior to the sacs in this view.

Clinical case resolution: Dog in respiratory distress

The dog at the beginning of the chapter was in significant respiratory distress. He was panting, trying to shed carbon dioxide. An orthopneic position is one in which the animal stands with his head down and front legs spread widely apart. This position requires less work on the part of the muscles of inhalation. Moving slowly helps him decrease metabolic activity and, thus, the need for oxygen.

In auscultating this animal, we find that breath sounds are diminished. Even though he is breathing rapidly, the air is not finding its way through the respiratory tract. Diminished breath sounds are usually associated with lower respiratory tract disease.

Radiography reveals that the animal has cardiomegaly and local inflammation of the lungs. These problems are commonly found together. One must take great care in positioning an animal with dyspnea for radiography. Having him lie down or stand in such a way as to increase respiratory effort is worse for the animal than not being able to get a good radiograph.

Review questions

1 What is vital capacity?

2 What is physiological dead space?

3 Define V/Q mismatch.

4 What is a chemoreceptor (as it relates to the respiratory system)?

5 True or false: Inserting an endotracheal (breathing) tube that is too long prior to surgery will not affect dead space but will have an impact on gas permeability of the alveolus.

6 What is the word for the collapse or a lung or lung lobe?

7 What does a hemoglobin/oxygen dissociation curve show us?

8 What do high levels of carbon dioxide do to blood pH?

9 Is exhalation in the dog and cat normally active or passive?

10 Which part of the bird's respiratory system expands and contracts?

Chapter **24** Reproductive Physiology

Clinical case: The howling feline

The owner of a female intact (capable of reproduction, not spayed) cat comes in describing a number of symptoms her young cat has recently developed. They include lordosis (arching of the back) and vocalizations that resemble howling. The cat has also been very restless. The client is quite concerned and believes the cat may be sick, although the cat is eating and otherwise seems to be fine. A discussion of reproductive physiology will help us explain the problem.

Introduction

There is a strong connection between the survivability of a species and its ability to bear viable young on a consistent basis. The combination of physical and chemical changes that occur in order for fertilization, pregnancy, and birth to occur in mammals has some things in common across species. There is much more

variety in lizards and avians, for example. However, the clinician in small animal practice will be well served by investigation of mammalian reproduction.

A cascade of events

The reproductive system depends on a wide variety of secretions and hormones in order to function. This system develops during youth but undergoes physical changes with aging. Hormonal ebb and flow also follows not only seasonal but also age-related cycles.

The series of events preceding and following ovulation are known as the estrous cycle. Estrus (note that the spelling of the noun is different from the spelling of the adjective) is the part of the cycle that denotes the time of female sexual receptivity to the male. It is also known as "heat." The only species that has a cycle that occurs every month, year-round, is the primate. That cycle is referred to as menstrual rather than estrous. The word "menstrual" comes from the root word for month, while the word "estrous" refers to one of the major reproductive hormones, estrogen.

Anatomy and Physiology for Veterinary Technicians and Nurses: A Clinical Approach, First Edition. Robin Sturtz and Lori Asprea.
© 2012 John Wiley & Sons, Inc. Published 2012 by John Wiley & Sons, Inc.

The female

The combination of the ovum (egg) produced by the female and the sperm (fertilizing agent) produced by the male forms the basis of the developing embryo. There are some mammals that are born with sets of both male and female reproductive organs. These animals are sterile (cannot reproduce). This is not true for all species, however; a single clown fish can produce both ova and sperm that are viable (lead to a newborn).

The ovary is the cranial-most part of the female reproductive system in dogs and cats. When a puppy or kitten is born, she has all of the ova (egg cells) she will ever have. Whether she mates or not, there will be a steady decrease in the number of ova available throughout life. As a result, fertility decreases over time.

The ovarian or estrous cycle refers to the series of physical and hormonal changes that occur from one estrus to the next. The cycle has four parts. Proestrus is the series of chemical and structural changes that prepare the animal for ovulation. It includes the growth of the follicle, under the influence of rising levels of estrogen. The follicle is the round "cushion" within which the ovum sits. Follicles might be seen as a protrusion from the ovary, like a blister, during ovariohysterectomy (spay) surgery if the surgery takes place during this part of the cycle. Proestrus is the time during which there may be bloody discharge from the vagina.

Estrus, as mentioned above, is the part of the cycle that is literally dominated by the female's receptivity to the male. From a hormonal standpoint, a cascade of events takes place. A peak level of estrogen leads to a surge of luteinizing hormone (LH), which, in turn, stimulates a sharp increase in progesterone levels. The level of LH declines so rapidly that it is actually back down to its resting level before the estrus phase is over. Estrus is associated with ovulation.

Progesterone (which is produced in the adrenal gland and by the placenta in the pregnant animal) continues to rise through diestrus, the next phase in the cycle. Estrogen (manufactured in the adrenal gland and the ovary) continues to decrease. If the animal were to become pregnant, the presence of progesterone would help maintain the pregnancy. If the animal does not become pregnant, the cycle enters anestrus. Anestrus is basically a time of reproductive system inactivity.

Hormonal control

A closer look at the hormones involved in the reproductive cycle will be helpful. Most of the hormones controlling the progression of steps through the ovarian cycle come from the pituitary. In particular, the anterior pituitary produces follicle-stimulating hormone (FSH), LH, and prolactin. The latter is associated with the production of milk. The posterior pituitary produces oxytocin. We have discussed oxytocin in its connection to milk letdown. It is also produced as the time of parturition nears. Its effect is to increase the contraction of the muscles of the uterine wall so that the puppy or kitten can be propelled out into the world.

Some of the hormones involved come from the tissues of the reproductive tract itself. Specifically, the ovary produces estrogen and testosterone, steroid compounds that provide an internal signal for the hypothalamus to monitor. If the animal does become pregnant, the membrane that grows around the infant will also produce these hormones. This membrane is known as the placenta.

As the ovum begins to grow, it is important that the follicle around it continue to develop. FSH is released from the pituitary in response to the appearance and early growth of the follicle. In addition to this stimulus, the cells of the follicle itself can take androgens such as testosterone and convert them to estrogen. As both are steroids, their chemical structure is not dissimilar, and the conversion is thus possible.

Estrogen helps the follicle to grow, providing a good environment for the ovum. In addition, the early follicle adds receptors for FSH, furthering its stimulation to grow. However, as estrogen levels in the follicle continue to rise, the presence of receptors to LH increases. With more LH receptors, the follicle is more sensitive to this hormone, which eventually causes the follicle to open and release the ovum into the reproductive tract.

Once the follicle collapses, it is referred to as a corpus luteum. The corpus luteum is still viable for a time, and in fact has an important role to play in the reproductive cycle. The corpus luteum produces progesterone, which prepares the uterus for pregnancy. This is called the luteal phase of the estrous cycle. In the absence of pregnancy, Prostaglandin F2 alpha (PGF2a) causes disruption of the corpus luteum, and the remnant of the follicle becomes fibrous tissue. New follicles will start to form, and the process repeats.

Diestrus is, as noted above, the stage after estrus. The production of progesterone is a part of the luteal phase of the cycle. If the animal has mated successfully, endocrine signals from the developing embryo will cause the corpus luteum to persist and continue pumping out progesterone. If there has been no mating (or mating has been unsuccessful, perhaps related to fertility issues), the corpus luteum will regress upon itself. This occurs during diestrus.

The canine estrous cycle lasts approximately 21 days, with the actual period of estrus a matter of days to a week (approximately; there are individual variations). Canines go through cycles twice a year.

During anestrus, the reproductive system undergoes little, if any, activity. Progesterone levels are very low, and other hormones, while present, do not undergo fluctuations.

A notable feature of the feline reproductive cycle is that the cat is a stimulated (or induced) ovulator; that is, the stimulation for the release of the oocyte from the follicle is in large part the act of copulation itself. While most mammals "automatically" ovulate, at which point they are in estrus, felines do not ovulate until they mate. There is still a follicle, and estrogen levels have to be at a certain point for the ovulation to occur. However, the corpus luteum does not form (in response to LH) until after copulation.

Felines produce a number of follicles at a time. In the absence of mating, these follicles will involute. What occurs is a series of follicular growth and collapse that persists over a number of days. Given that a number of follicles are available, and that the act of mating provokes ovulation, it is quite possible to have a litter of kittens in which some have different sires.

Briefly, then, a series of hormonal changes leads to the growth of the follicle (FSH) and its discharge of the egg (LH). Estrogen stimulates the onset of estrus and rises again when birth is imminent. Progesterone prepares the uterus for pregnancy.

Prolactin, one of the pituitary hormones, is associated with maintaining the corpus luteum. In other words, it continues the ovary's production of progesterone, which maintains the pregnancy. If prolactin is released in the absence of fertilization, the result is something called pseudopregnancy. Under this condition, the animal will exhibit the behavioral signs of pregnancy but will not actually be carrying an embryo.

Many domestic animals are seasonally polyestrous. That means that they have more than one estrous cycle, but only at certain times of the year. Felines are a good example of this.

Other factors affecting the estrous cycle

Puberty is defined as the time the female begins to ovulate, or the time a male can produce enough sperm to impregnate a female. The first ovulation does not generally result in pregnancy even if mating occurs. The onset of puberty is about 6 months for dogs and cats, although it can occur months later in larger-breed dogs. Poor nutrition and certain disease states can delay the onset of puberty.

Photoperiod also has an effect on the estrous cycle. Longer hours of daylight in a 24-hour period are one of the triggers of the development of the follicle and the growth of the oocyte. Interestingly, sheep actually are more prone to be in estrus during times when daylight hours are fewer.

Ovarian activity can be affected by lactation. In some species, such as swine, lactation actually suppresses activity in the ovary, and successful mating cannot take place until after piglets are weaned.

Pheromones play a role in the estrous cycle. In a kennel or cattery, male pheromone will often cause the estrous cycles of the animals to become synchronous. In return, female pheromone will increase the male's desire to mate.

During feline estrus, the widely fluctuating hormones can be a cause of unusual behaviors. Arching of the back and increased vocalizations are some of them. These behaviors also serve to "advertise" the female's receptivity to any males in the area.

The male

The production of sperm is the province of the testicles. As the sperm continue along the deferent duct, various fluids are added, and the resulting solution is called semen. Many of the same hormones discussed in conjunction with the female will be discussed in conjunction with the male.

Spermatogenesis is the process of producing sperm. It must occur at a specific temperature in mammals. However, that temperature does vary by species. The testicles are extra-abdominal (on the outside of the body) in dogs and cats, intra-abdominal or retractable in other species. All of these structural differences exist to ensure that the production of viable sperm is possible. The more favorable the temperature, the better the quality of the sperm.

The production of sperm begins in the seminiferous tubules, microscopic channels within the testicle. The process of producing sperm cells is under the direction of LH. FSH also plays a role here. FSH stimulates some of the cells that assist in building the spermatozoa (sperm cells) to produce a small amount of estrogen.

As the spermatozoa continue to develop, they begin to move through another series of tubules until they reach the epididymis. As they move along the epididymis, they have extra time in which to mature. Eventually, they reach the ductus deferens, which brings the sperm cells along through the penis. The sperm are actually discharged from the urethra as the deferent duct meets up with the urethra proximal to leaving the body.

The process of erection is related to the presence of cavernous tissue. This tissue has many hollows that allow it to stiffen when filled with blood. Ejaculation is the process of expelling semen from the body. These actions are under parasympathetic and sympathetic nervous system control, respectively. There are other factors as well, including psychobehavioral ones, although these are less common than in humans. Hormonal imbalances can affect the ability of the male to produce and/or discharge semen. The proper word for the introduction of ejaculate into a female is intromission.

Oxytocin is released in males in response to copulation. The muscle contraction in the reproductive tract that is caused helps move the sperm along into the more cranial parts of the tract.

While in the reproductive tract of the female, the sperm begins to undergo a process called capacitation. This involves the release of enzymes that allow the sperm to penetrate the ovum. Spermatozoa will try to implant in a number of places on the ovum. Once one has penetrated the ovum, the membrane will not allow other sperm to enter. As there are multiple ova, the number of spermatozoa that find an ovum in which to achieve entry is greater than in primates, who generally only produce one or two ova.

Fertilization and pregnancy

Once the ovum is fertilized, it is called a zygote. Each sperm cell or ovum has only half the normal number of chromosomes an adult cell has. It is only when the zygote is formed that the chromosomes join together.

A significant difference between dogs and cats has to do with the location of fertilization and pregnancy. Ovum and sperm actually come together in the oviduct. As they begin to work together, they move slightly caudally to rest in the uterine horns. The growth of the embryo and fetus occurs in the uterine horns, not in the body of the uterus.

The newly fertilized ovum will begin to divide itself to make new cells, using the genetic material of the sperm as well as its own. At this point, it does not increase in size. Until the time it implants itself in the walls of the uterus, it is referred to as a zygote. Once it implants itself, it is called an embryo. Once it begins to show differentiated organs, it is referred to as a fetus.

The small cluster of cells that will become the fetus implants in the endometrium, which is the inner lining, of the uterine horn. As the zygote settles into the uterine lining, a membrane begins to develop around it. This membrane is called the placenta. Nutrients and oxygen-rich blood will be provided to the embryo through this membrane. The placenta is connected to the embryo by way of a stalk-like structure called the umbilicus.

Note that the embryo/fetus does not breathe air but receives oxygen through the bloodstream. As a result, there is no need for blood to circulate through the lungs as it journeys around the fetus's body. Blood entering one side of the heart is immediately shunted to the other side of the heart, bypassing the lungs altogether. The reader will recall structures like the ductus arteriosus and foramen ovale that help blood pass through the fetal heart without circling through the lungs.

There is tremendous variation in the location and complexity of the attachment of the placenta to the uterus. The structure is actually more complicated in large animals than it is in dogs and cats, and even less complicated in primates. The attachment of the placenta to the uterus in cattle is so firm that the placenta occasionally will not be expelled after the calf is born. This condition is called retained placenta.

Under normal circumstances, the pregnancy of the dog or cat is approximately 63 days. This contrasts favorably with the gestation period (length of pregnancy) of the elephant, which is approximately 21 months.

The dog or cat generally has four to six newborns in a litter. However, this number varies, particularly in the case of larger dogs. It is of great concern if only one or two animals are born, and the mother should be checked carefully for any signs of retained fetuses or other problems.

Parturition

As mentioned earlier, progesterone helps keep the pregnancy viable. As the size of the fetus and the weight of the uterus reach a certain point, a number of changes occur. The amount of cortisol in the fetus rises and triggers secretion of estrogen. The rise in estrogen level, in turn, causes the release of oxytocin from the maternal pituitary.

Oxytocin causes contraction of the uterine muscles, leading each fetus to gradually move toward the body of the uterus. From there, the fetus is pushed toward the exit of the body. At this point, the cervix has relaxed enough that the puppy or kitten can slip through. Note that the muscle contraction will continue past the point that the last fetus is delivered. This will make sure that all placental material has been expelled as well.

Release of prostaglandin from the uterus eventually leads to regression of the corpus luteum and decline in progesterone levels. The placenta produces a hormone called relaxin. Relaxin, as the name implies, decreases the stiffness in the muscles and ligaments surrounding the pelvis, easing the passage of the newborn through the birth canal (vagina).

Although not directly related to the birth process itself, another hormonal event at this time is the release of prolactin from the pituitary gland. The rise in prolactin levels that accompanies pregnancy stimulates the production of colostrum. As mentioned in an earlier chapter, prolactin continues to stimulate the production of milk once the colostrum has been used up. It is joined in this effort by growth hormone. Milk production does not occur during pregnancy, in part because of the levels of progesterone and estrogen, which have an inhibitory effect on lactation.

Clinical case resolution: The howling feline

It should now be apparent that the cat described at the beginning of this chapter is in heat. The exaggerated behaviors she exhibits are in response to the changing hormonal composition of the bloodstream and its effect on local tissues, as well as the changes within the ovary. The behaviors are unrelieved until ovulation is stimulated by copulation. The nature of stimulated ovulation gives rise to the possibility of multiple sires for a given litter (although it is technically possible to have more than one sire for a litter of puppies). If a number of males copulate with a potential mate while she is in heat, she will ovulate each time, and thus the kittens in that litter may have different genetic material.

Review questions

1 Define estrus.
2 What are the four stages of the estrous cycle?
3 What is the corpus luteum?
4 True or false: The FSH is found in females but not in males.
5 LH is associated with the bursting open of the follicle, which is accompanied by a steep rise in what hormone?
6 True or false: There is no hormonal activity during anestrus.
7 What hormone produced in the fetus triggers the release of estrogen as parturition approaches?
8 What connects the placenta to the embryo?
9 What is capacitation of sperm?
10 What does stimulated ovulation mean? Is it found in dogs, cats, or both?

Appendix **1** Dissection Notes

A few suggestions for dissecting the specimen cleanly so that it can be easily studied:

The use of clean instruments is essential. Follow instructor directions regarding handling sharps. Scalpel blades can be reused in laboratory dissection, as there is no fear of contaminating the animal, but a new blade should be put in place when the first one becomes dull.

Scalpel blades make cuts (incise) quite easily, with minimal pressure, when the blade is new. For tougher tissue, like skin, the scalpel blade should be used, but be careful not to press down hard or use a sawing motion. It is easy to cut down through tissue one wishes to examine later if too much force is applied.

For material like smaller muscles and internal organs, a scissor is usually sufficient. This avoids cutting through too many layers at once. In separating layers of muscle, or organs from fascia, it is best to use the blunt dissector in your kit rather than a sharp instrument. Again, the goal is to avoid destruction of the organs or tissue surrounding the area on which one is working.

When looking at layers of musculature, work from the superficial layer to the deeper layer. Once a superficial muscle has been excavated, use a scissor to cut across the midline of the muscle, rather than separating it from the bone or joint. This will allow you to reflect (fold back) the superficial muscle and to see what lies underneath. The superficial muscle can later be folded back into place for later study.

Hollow organs, such as intestines, stomach, and urinary bladder, may still contain digested material or urine, respectively. Be careful in incising these organs, and keep one's face as far away from the area being worked on as possible.

Most preserved specimens contain formalin, a solution that is 10% formaldehyde. Formaldehyde can cause injury or illness, and handling any fluid materials within the animal should be done with utmost care. The use of goggles is highly recommended. The use of examination gloves is essential. Nitrile gloves are preferred for working with formalin as they are less permeable to formaldehyde than latex. In addition, some people are allergic to latex, which makes nitrile a better alternative.

As is true in any laboratory, the use of protective clothing and closed-toe shoes is required. Be sure to change clothes before returning home so that chemicals or organic materials are not transported along.

Anatomy and Physiology for Veterinary Technicians and Nurses: A Clinical Approach, First Edition. Robin Sturtz and Lori Asprea.
© 2012 John Wiley & Sons, Inc. Published 2012 by John Wiley & Sons, Inc.

Appendix 2 The Cranial Nerves

Number	Name	Related to
I	Olfactory	sense of smell
II	Optic	visual images
III	Oculomotor	eye movement
IV	Trochlear	eye movement
V	Trigeminal	facial sensation, movement of many muscles of the head
VI	Abducent	eye movement
VII	Facial	movement of facial muscles sense of taste
VIII	Vestibulocochlear	balance and sound reception
IX	Glossopharyngeal	movement in tongue and throat salivation, sense of taste
X	Vagus	autonomic nervous system
XI	Accessory	muscles of the throat and chest
XII	Hypoglossal	muscles of the tongue

Most students use a mnemonic device to remember the names of the nerves. One that uses the first letter of the name of each nerve as the first letter of a word in a sentence is:

On Old Olympus the Truth Touches (a) Few Very Good, Very Accepting Hearts. (olfactory, optic, etc.)

A search of the Internet will yield many other choices, or the reader can construct a new one.

Most of the cranial nerves arise from the brain stem or the medulla oblongata. The accessory nerve has some fibers that arise from the cervical spinal cord.

The vagus is the longest of the cranial nerves. The trigeminal nerve has a relatively large diameter and has a number of prominent branches.

Anatomy and Physiology for Veterinary Technicians and Nurses: A Clinical Approach, First Edition. Robin Sturtz and Lori Asprea.
© 2012 John Wiley & Sons, Inc. Published 2012 by John Wiley & Sons, Inc.

Appendix **3** Selected Muscle Origins and Insertions

From origin to insertion

Masseter: zygomatic arch to mandible

Pectorals: sternum to humerus

Deltoid: scapula to deltoid tuberosity of humerus

Trapezius: neck and cranial thoracic vertebrae to spine of the scapula

Serratus ventralis: cervical vertebrae (and cranial ribs, for thoracic part of muscle) to scapula

Supraspinatus: scapula to humerus

Biceps brachii: scapula to radius

Extensor carpi radialis: lateral epicondyle (area just proximal to the condyle) of humerus to metacarpus

Lateral ulnar: lateral epicondyle of humerus to metacarpal V

Superficial digital flexor: medial condyle of the humerus to the palmar surface of the middle phalanges

Latissimus dorsi: thoracolumbar spine to humerus

Internal and external abdominal obliques: ribs to linea alba

Middle gluteal: ilium to greater trochanter of femur

Biceps femoris: ischium to patella, tibia, and calcaneus

Tensor fasciae latae: pelvis to lateral femoral fascia

Quadriceps: actually four different heads in the femoral area that converge at the patellar tendon, which contains the patella itself

Biceps femoris: ischiatic tuberosity to patella, tibia, and calcaneus

Semitendinosus: ischiatic tuberosity to tibial crest and calcaneus

Semimembranosus: ischiatic tuberosity to medial femur and tibia

Sartorius: ilium to medial stifle

Gracilis: pelvic (pubic) symphysis to medial stifle and calcaneus

Cranial tibial: proximal tibia to plantar surface of metatarsals I and II

Gastrocnemius: distocaudal femur to calcaneus

Coccygeus: ischium to tail

Levator ani: pelvis to tail

Anatomy and Physiology for Veterinary Technicians and Nurses: A Clinical Approach, First Edition. Robin Sturtz and Lori Asprea.
© 2012 John Wiley & Sons, Inc. Published 2012 by John Wiley & Sons, Inc.

Answers

Chapter 1

1 Medial: toward the midline
 Rostral: toward the front of the face
 Dorsal: upward
2 The thoracic limb
3 Palmar
4 False
5 The anatomy of the parts of an organ or area compared to the whole.

Chapter 2

1 Dermis and epidermis
2 Anal, interdigital, suborbital
3 Yes
4 Dermatophytes
5 Digital pad
6 A condition where the layers making up the hoof are separated by inflammation, leading to severe pain
7 Tactile hairs are thicker and stiffer.
8 Antlers shed, horns do not.
9 Ringworm
10 Shortening the primary contour feathers

Chapter 3

1 Scapula, pelvis, ribs
2 Diaphysis
3 Three, except in the dewclaw, which has two
4 Atlas
5 Sesamoid

Chapter 4

1 Pennate, spindle, strap, sphincter
2 Skeletal muscle is associated with voluntary movement, smooth muscle with involuntary movement.
3 Superficial and deep pectoral muscles
4 It runs caudal to cranial from origin to insertion.
5 External and internal abdominal oblique muscles
6 Semimembranosis and semitendinosis. We need to identify them to be sure we know where the sciatic nerve is.
7 Crus; gastrocnemius and cranial tibial
8 Dorsal
9 Infraspinatus
10 Biceps brachii
11 An aponeurosis that joins the superficial abdominal muscles
12 Lateral thorax, deep to the lastissimus dorsi

Chapter 5

1 Metacarpophalangeal
2 Nuchal
3 Capsule, collateral ligaments, cranial and caudal cruciate ligaments, menisci, fat pad, patella
4 Synovial, fibrous, cartilaginous
5 White or pink
6 Stifle, TMJ, shoulder
7 A suture is an immobile joint on the skull; a symphysis is a fibrous joint elsewhere on the body, which may flex slightly.
8 A fibrocarilagenous lip that surrounds a part of the joint, present on the bone; acetabulum
9 A test to check the cranial cruciate ligament, checking to see if the tibia moves abnormally compared to the femur
10 Atlantoaxial

Anatomy and Physiology for Veterinary Technicians and Nurses: A Clinical Approach, First Edition. Robin Sturtz and Lori Asprea.
© 2012 John Wiley & Sons, Inc. Published 2012 by John Wiley & Sons, Inc.

Chapter 6

1 Radial and median
2 Collection of nerve bodies outside of the brain
3 Spinal accessory
4 Myelin
5 Ischiatic nerve
6 Epidural space
7 Foramen magnum
8 Cisterna magna or lumbar puncture
9 Auriculopalpebral
10 Fasciculus

Chapter 7

1 Renal medulla
2 Hilus
3 True
4 Dorsal
5 It curves around before it exits the body, leaving it vulnerable to obstruction.

Chapter 8

1 Pericardium
2 Left ventricle
3 Aortic bulb
4 Pulmonary trunk or pulmonary artery
5 Celiac artery
6 False
7 Arterioles
8 Cranial vena cava
9 It stores red blood cells.
10 Popliteal

Chapter 9

1 Palatoglossal arch
2 Dog
3 Left cranial
4 Duodenum
5 Ascending, transverse, and descending
6 the pancreas has a duct that opens into the duodenum.
7 Reticulum, rumen, omasum, abomasum
8 cecum

Chapter 10

1 Pituitary gland
2 Neck (near larynx)
3 Contributes to wake/sleep cycle, is light sensitive
4 Craniomedial to the kidney
5 Pancreas (specifically, islets of Langerhans); yes; digestion

Chapter 11

1 Pleura
2 Cartilage
3 Philtrum
4 Seven
5 Glottis

Chapter 12

1 Queen
2 Ovary
3 Infundibulum
4 horn of the uterus
5 Yes
6 False (it is ventral to the rectum)
7 An S-shaped curve, present in the penis of some ruminants

Chapter 13

1 Phospholipid
2 No
3 Breaking of ATP bonds releases energy.
4 False
5 No
6 It refers to the balance of addition and subtraction of oxygen during chemical reactions.

Chapter 14

1 The transfer of cooler temperature to the skin from nearby cold air
2 An animal whose core temperature depends on ambient temperature, and thus is not constant
3 Arrector pili
4 Vibrissae
5 Sweat
6 An odor that only animals of the same species can sense
7 Horns are permanent, while antlers are shed and regrow every year.
8 Dog, cat, horse

Chapter 15

1 False
2 Yes, it would be in the same position. Bones grow from the ends, not the middle.
3 Cartilage
4 periosteum
5 Mature, fully developed bone
6 They are cells that break down bone cells.
7 No
8 Hyaline cartilage
9 True

Chapter 16

1 True
2 acetylcholine
3 sarcoplasmic reticulum
4 autonomic, norepinephrine
5 Smooth muscle
6 Smooth muscle

Chapter 17

1 Gustatory
2 The adjective associated with the sense of balance and orientation in space
3 False
4 Middle ear
5 The reflective layer of the choroid that enhances the brightness of light
6 Sclera
7 True
8 An area of soft tissue that makes odors stronger when air is pulled across the organ

Chapter 18

1 Underdevelopment of the cerebellum
2 −75 mV
3 As a demyelinated area, the action potential can jump across it and speed up.
4 the electrical charge of the cell is less negative.
5 A gap between one neuron and another
6 The stimulation would continue, and the response would be continuous, even to the point of damaging the organism.
7 A voltage-gated channel is one that opens in response to a change in electrical charge; a ligand-gated channel is one that opens because either the transmitter or an accompanying molecule fits into the channel specifically.
8 Speeds it up
9 The brain and the spinal cord
10 The patellar or "knee jerk" reflex

Chapter 19

1 Glomerulus, proximal convoluted tubule, loop of Henle (ascending loop and descending loop), distal tubule, collecting duct
2 If the material coming out of the glomerulus is the same as the material that exits the kidney, the nephron has not changed it at all and therefore is not working.
3 False
4 The kidney produces a hormone, EPO, that signals the bone marrow to produce more red blood cells.
5 Makes it resorb more water
6 False
7 True

Chapter 20

1 Stroke volume times heart rate
2 The heartbeat would be unorganized or irregular.
3 Starling's law says that stroke volume increases as preload increases.
4 ventricles
5 afterload
6 pressure or stretching in the blood vessels
7 When the heartbeat and the pulse of the arteries are not synchronous
8 It decreases.
9 Yes
10 Veins

Chapter 21

1 Aggression/defense, amplifying sound, thermoregulation
2 To increase the surface area for digestion
3 It comes into the digestive tract at the duodenum and helps digest fats.
4 Resorb water
5 Rise
6 Abomasum

Chapter 22

1 Fall
2 Uterine contraction, milk letdown; causes smooth muscle to constrict
3 A series of events that lead to the endocrine system decreasing the output of a hormone when its blood levels get too high
4 Yes, because they inhibit the work of fibroblasts, which are part of the healing process.
5 The endocrine cells within the pancreas that produce insulin
6 The glucose levels would rise.
7 Adrenal medulla
8 No, they are secreted directly into the bloodstream.
9 Stimulates gluconeogenesis, glycogen breakdown, and increases serum glucose levels

Chapter 23

1 The amount of air that moves in and out in one breath cycle
2 The amount of inactive area in the alveoli during respiration plus the amount of space that does not actually exchange gases (usually, from the nose to the main bronchus)
3 When the tidal volume does not match up with the amount of perfusion in the alveoli, and gas exchange is inefficient
4 An area of cells that are sensitive to blood pH
5 False
6 Atelectasis
7 How easily oxygen can leave the hemoglobin that is carrying it so that it can enter the cells of the body
8 Decrease it

9 Passive
10 Air sacs

Chapter 24

1 When the female is sexually receptive to the male
2 Proestrus, estrus, diestrus, anestrus
3 The follicle after it has ruptured
4 False

5 Progesterone
6 False
7 Cortisol
8 Umbilicus
9 A chemical change that allows the sperm to penetrate the ovum.
10 A condition in which the animal does not ovulate until copulation occurs. It is found in cats but in not dogs.

Glossary

Action potential   The wave of electrical energy that is directed toward a target cell or organ.

Acute onset   A problem or disease that appears suddenly.

Allergen   A material that causes a hypersensitivity (allergic) response.

Antebrachium   The part of the thoracic limb from the elbow to the carpus.

Articular surface   The surface of a bone that is within the joint.

Aspirate   To bring anything other than air into the trachea; also, to remove liquid or other soft material from a body structure by way of a needle or catheter.

Atelectasis   The collapse of one or more lobes of the lung.

ATP (adenosine triphosphate)   A product of chemical reactions that liberate a substantial amount of energy for cells to use.

Auscult   Listen; particularly, to listen to the chest or abdomen in order to assess the status of organs within it.

Axilla   The area ventral to the shoulder joint ("armpit").

Biopsy   Surgically taking a sample of tissue so that it can be analyzed.

Brachium   The part of the thoracic limb from the shoulder to the elbow.

Calculus   When referring to medicine, it means a concretion of minerals or other hard materials, informally called a "stone." Calculi (plural) are often found in the urinary bladder, and less commonly in the kidney and gallbladder.

Canthus   An angle, particularly one where two structures meet. The lateral canthus of the eye is the spot on the side of the head where the upper and lower eyelids meet; the medial canthus is the equivalent spot toward the midline.

Caudal direction   Toward the tail.

Cavity   An opening, usually fairly large, within which are other organs. The major cavities of the body are the thoracic (chest) and peritoneal (abdomen) cavities. Also, a defect in a tooth.

Cellular respiration   The way that a cell creates energy to manufacture proteins or other substances needed for normal performance.

Cervid   The family of hoofed stock including deer.

Ciliated cell   A cell with one or more hairlike structures on its surface.

Compact bone   Mature bone that has great strength.

Continent/incontinent   The ability to urinate or defecate at the appropriate place and time is called continence. An animal that cannot control when or where they urinate or defecate is said to be incontinent.

Cranial direction   Toward the head.

Chronic   A condition or disease that continues over time; can be intermittent or steady.

Cortex   The outer layer of some organs, such as the adrenal gland and the kidney; also, the part of the brain encompassing the areas related to higher/integrative thinking.

Cytoplasm   The liquid portion of a somatic cell.

Anatomy and Physiology for Veterinary Technicians and Nurses: A Clinical Approach, First Edition. Robin Sturtz and Lori Asprea.
© 2012 John Wiley & Sons, Inc. Published 2012 by John Wiley & Sons, Inc.

Distal   Further away from the trunk of the body.

Distensible   Expands and contracts easily, as the urinary bladder.

Dorsal   Upward (directional term).

Dyspnea   Difficulty breathing.

Ectopic   In an abnormal or unusual place, such as thyroid tissue, that appears in the chest instead of in the gland itself.

Electrolyte   Molecules such as potassium, calcium, and sodium, which are capable of becoming ions (losing or gaining an electron).

Endocrine organ   An organ that produces hormones, chemicals that stimulate the production of hormones, or neurotransmitters. Usually ductless.

Endoplasmic reticulum   The energy storage component of a somatic cell.

Endotracheal   Within the trachea; often used in the phrase "endotracheal tube," which is a tube inserted through the mouth down into the trachea, used for breathing when an animal is under anesthesia.

Enteric   Referring specifically to the small intestine.

Estrous cyle   The series of chemical events that lead to ovulation and either pregnancy or the end of the chemical cycle.

Fascicle (plural: fasciculi)   A collection of muscle fibers into one bundle; also, a collection of nerve fibers into one bundle.

Fasciculation   Localized muscle twitching.

Fenestrated   Has windows or pores in its walls; often refers to blood vessels.

Gait   The way an animal walks or runs; an abnormal gait would imply limping or not being able to coordinate movements of the limbs.

Gestation period   The amount of time the animal is normally pregnant.

Homeostasis   The level of performance the body needs to maintain in order to continue normal function; applies to many things, but particularly to keeping a normal energy level and pH balance.

Hormone   A substance that changes metabolic function or stimulates the neurological system; generally discharged directly into the bloodstream.

Iatrogenic   The description of a disease or dysfunction that occurs as the unexpected result of medical treatment; a medical problem caused by treatment for another disorder.

Ingesta   Material that has been taken into the digestive tract at least as far as the esophagus. Note that this material is not necessarily composed of nutrients.

Interstitial tissue/interstice   Small spaces or areas of connective tissue within organs or between them, excluding the major body cavities like the thoracic and peritoneal cavities.

Lobe   A separate but connected section of a larger organ; for example, both the liver and the lung are composed of a series of "flaps" called lobes.

Lumen   The hollow part of the inside of a tube; the luminal surface is the layer that forms the boundary of the inside of the hole.

Luxate   The act of moving out of a normal position, temporarily or permanently; usually refers to bones or joint components.

Mediastinum   The space between the left and right lungs, enclosing the heart as well as sections of the trachea and esophagus, in addition to nerves and blood vessels.

Medulla   The inner section of some organs, including the adrenal gland and kidneys.

Metabolism   A series of activities that lead to the continuation of basic bodily systems such as digestion, respiration, cardiovascular circulation, and cellular activity, or the rate of speed or strength of response of these functions.

Minute ventilation   The amount of air moved in and out of the body in 1 minute; in other words, tidal volume times breaths per minute.

Mnemonic device   A way of remembering things by using another (presumably, easier to recall) word or letter to represent each item.

Olfactory   Having to do with the sense of smell.

Oncotic pressure   The molecular "attraction" that causes osmotic movement.

Orchiectomy   Surgical removal of the testicles; neuter.

Orthopneic   A posture an animal assumes when it is having trouble breathing, involving the thoracic limbs spread apart, back hunched, and head down.

Osmosis   The movement of liquid toward an area of higher concentration of solutes.

Osteon   A circular structure containing cells that are the main support for compact bone.

Ovarian cyle   The amount of time between estrous cycles.

Ovariohysterectomy   Surgical removal of the ovaries and uterus; spay.

Parturition   The act of giving birth.

pH   A measure of acidity/alkalinity. A low pH means having an acidic quality, and a high pH an alkaline quality. Normal pH in mammals is usually different from that of water, which is 7.0.

Phlebotomy   The removal of blood from a vein or artery by way of a needle.

Pinna   The visible, cartilaginous part of the outer ear.

Polydactyly   Having more than the usual number of digits; a polydactyl dog has 21 or more digits, a cat 19 or more.

Prehension   The act of grasping something.

Pronate   Move a distal limb from palmar/plantar surface up to palmar/plantar surface down; the equivalent of slapping the palm on the ground.

Pruritic   Itchy.

Saline   A solution of salt and water.

Sarcolemma   The membrane (border) of a muscle cell.

Sarcoplasma   The liquid portion of a muscle cell.

Sarcoplasmic reticulum   The energy storage container of a muscle cell.

Sesamoid   Having the appearance of a sesame seed; usually refers to small bones that appear in association with joints of the limbs and help cushion ligaments or tendons as they move.

Spinal column, divisions of   From cranial to caudal, cervical, thoracic, lumbar, sacral, caudal.

Spinal cord   The thick cable of nerve fibers that runs from the brain to the cauda equina.

Supinate   On the distal limb, moving the palmar/plantar surface of the limb so that it is facing upward.

Tidal volume   The total amount of air moved in one breath.

Trunk of the body   The thorax and abdomen taken as one unit; the body of the animal minus the head, tail and limbs.

Vascularization   How well supplied an area is with blood vessels; neovascularization refers to the formation of new blood vessels in an area.

Ventral   Downward (directional term; applies only to the trunk and head).

Viscera   The internal organs of the abdomen and thorax.

Zoonotic disease   A condition that humans can develop from contact with an infected animal or animal product.

References

Bibliography

Akers R, Denbow D. *Anatomy and Physiology of Domestic Animals*, 1st ed. John Wiley & Sons, Ames, IA, 2008.

Cunningham J (ed.) *Textbook of Veterinary Physiology*, 3rd ed. Elsevier Health Sciences, St. Louis, MO, 2007.

Dyce K, Sack W, Wensing C. *Textbook of Veterinary Anatomy*, 2nd ed. W.B. Saunders Company, St. Louis, MO, 1996.

Feldman E, Nelson R. *Canine and Feline Endocrinology and Reproduction*, 3rd ed. Elsevier Health Sciences, St. Louis, MO, 2003.

Pasquini C, Spurgeon T, Pasquini S. *Anatomy of Domestic Animals*, 11th ed. SUDZ Publishing, Pilot Point, TX, 2007.

Reece W. *Functional Anatomy and Physiology of Domestic Animals*, 4th ed. Wiley-Blackwell, Ames, IA, 2009.

Stedman's Medical Dictionary, 27th ed. Lippincott, Williams and Wilkins, Philadelphia, 2000.

Further reading

Using anatomy for clinical purposes

Fowler M. *Restraint and Handling of Wild and Domestic Animals*, 2nd ed. John Wiley & Sons, Ames, IA, 2008.

Ballard B. *Restraint & Handling for Veterinary Technicians and Assistants*, 1st ed. Cengage Learning, Independence, KY, 2009.

Cheville N. *Introduction to Veterinary Pathology*, 3rd ed. John Wiley & Sons, Ames, IA, 2006.

Lavin L. *Radiography in Veterinary Technology*, 4th ed. Elsevier Health Sciences, St. Louis, MO, 2006.

DuPont G. *Atlas of Dental Radiography in Dogs and Cats*. Elsevier Health Sciences, St. Louis, MO, 2008.

Hyttel P. *Essentials of Domestic Animal Embryology*. Elsevier Health Sciences, St. Louis, MO, 2009.

Using anatomy and physiology for clinical purposes

Greene C. *Infectious Diseases of the Dog and Cat*, 3rd ed. (revised reprint). Elsevier Health Sciences, St. Louis, MO, 2006.

Hrapkiewicz K. *Clinical Laboratory Animal Medicine: An Introduction*, 3rd ed. John Wiley & Sons, Ames, IA, 2007.

And what every technologist should have

Stedman's Medical Dictionary, 27th ed. Featuring New Veterinary Medicine Insert With Over 45 Images and References, produced by Stedman's Lippincott Williams and Wilkins, Philadelphia, 2003.

Index